Choosing Nursing

Becoming a nurse is a life-changing process and making the decision to study nursing at university is the first step. This short guide will help you decide whether it is the right move for you, give you an idea of which field of nursing might suit you best and provide useful tips for making a successful application.

Outlining the academic and clinical support that students can expect during their study, the stresses that they may face, how placements work and the role of the NMC for student nurses, this book includes a wide range of testimonials from nursing students as well as practising nurses.

Most importantly, it shows what is unique about each of the different fields, which include children's, adult, mental health, learning disability and defence nursing. It also looks at what all of these areas have in common – what makes nursing nursing and what makes nursing special.

With a final section looking to the future, with tips for getting your first job and highlighting nursing opportunities around the globe, this is the must-have, no-nonsense career advice book for all those considering nursing as a career option or waiting to start their nursing course – or indeed for those nurses who are wishing to return to the nursing profession.

Cathy Poole has over 33 years' experience in health and education. She has held positions in adult orthopaedics, children's nursing, nursing management, the private sector and the higher education sector. Her main area of interest is renal nursing and she maintains her clinical professional development as a Bank Staff Nurse at a Children's Hospice.

Choosing Nursing

From application to offer and beyond

Edited by Cathy Poole

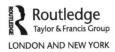
Routledge
Taylor & Francis Group

LONDON AND NEW YORK

First published 2015
by Routledge
2 Park Square, Milton Park, Abingdon, Oxon OX14 4RN

and by Routledge
711 Third Avenue, New York, NY 10017

Routledge is an imprint of the Taylor & Francis Group, an informa business

© 2015 selection and editorial material, C. Poole; individual chapters, the contributors

British Library Cataloguing-in-Publication Data
A catalogue record for this book is available from the British Library

Library of Congress Cataloging in Publication Data
Choosing nursing : from application to offer and beyond / edited by Cathy Poole.
    p. ; cm.
Includes bibliographical references and index.
I. Poole, Cathy, editor.
[DNLM: 1. Nursing. 2. Vocational Guidance. 3. Career Choice. WY 16.1]
RT82
610.7306'9—dc23   2014043970

ISBN: 978-0-415-53377-5 (hbk)
ISBN: 978-0-415-53378-2 (pbk)
ISBN: 978-0-203-11402-5 (ebk)

Typeset in Goudy
by Keystroke, Station Road, Codsall, Wolverhampton

To all those would-be nurses out there and to those of you who are already navigating your nursing career journey and, last but not least, to those of you who are returning to nursing practice to restart your nursing career voyage.

Good luck to each and every one of you.

Contents

18 Embarking on a journey of lifelong learning 173

TONY WHITTLE AND CATHY POOLE

Figures

FIGURE 5

Boxes

Foreword

I am delighted to be asked to write the foreword for a book which so elegantly complements existing literature aimed at individuals considering nursing as a career. I believe the content will help ensure that informed choices are made, whatever the decision. Uniquely, the following pages focus on assisting people to navigate in a logical way the complicated application process when either embarking for the first time on a career in nursing or when returning to practise after a break. Importantly, the text is realistic, practical and informative about the opportunities that exist within the four fields of practice described in Part 2: adult; children and young people; mental health; and learning disability. Defence nursing is also described.

I particularly like the quotes from existing students; they bring authority to the text alongside the personal experience of the chapter authors. Part 3 sets out the Nursing and Midwifery Council (NMC) standards for pre-registration nursing education, notably the professional and clinical competencies required: communication and interpersonal skills, decision making skills and the ability to lead, manage and work within a team. Most important of all, however, since the Independent Inquiry into care provided by Mid Staffordshire NHS Foundation Trust January 2005 – March 2009 are the professional values included in the NMC standards. The importance of appreciating the relevance of values at the beginning of a professional career in healthcare is now paramount as a consequence of the Inquiry findings. The skills and qualities needed to practise nursing well are further explored in Part 3. Of particular significance for me is the notion of trustworthiness, which is so important in securing public confidence in the profession.

Being a student is not easy. Being a nursing student can be particularly demanding at times. Part 4 therefore, which describes the kind of support students can expect and the strategies they can adopt, is I think both reassuring and a helpful framework for those who probably will have not encountered some of the scenarios previously. The book is realistic about the stresses students might face, which reinforces my view that the text is grounded and authentic.

The concluding section (Part 5) is about securing a job. The practical stance taken throughout the book is once again evident here. I think this section will assist the daunting task of finding suitable employment. The pace of change in healthcare, the rapidly expanding range of new technologies, and plethora of national policies is considerable, but the core of nursing remains the same, based on many of the values and skills outlined throughout the book. Students should be able to judge if their individual skills match the necessary skills and attributes highlighted prior to undertaking their pre-registration programme and again on completion when they are about to embark on a lifetime of learning. I began my career in 1967; I have loved every moment and regret no experience, although some have been tough. It would have been wonderful however to have had a clearer idea about what I was embarking on at the start! The 'six Cs' are mentioned in Part 4 as part of what a student can expect. I believe that one of them – Courage – is required by all who enter healthcare. It is a daunting task to care for people with complex needs, especially when resources are stretched. This book, however, helps prepare individuals to recognise this at an early stage but, importantly, alongside the many very real pleasures nursing can also bring.

Cathy Poole is to be commended on such a comprehensive and unique text. Many congratulations to all who have contributed to such a useful book.

Dame Elizabeth Fradd
DBE, RSCN, SRN, RM, HV Cert.

Preface

In order for you to be drawn into this book I want to tell you a little about myself. That way you will hopefully realise that I have the knowledge, skills and motivation to be an author with credibility.

When I was at school I found learning very difficult. I was not really able to read until I was about 11 years old and spelling was a real trauma. In all honesty I would have rather been climbing trees and building go-carts with my brother! So at parents' evenings the teachers would say to my mum and dad 'Ah well we cannot say what Cathy will achieve but whatever she does we know she will be happy.' Clearly therefore they had not got any real aspirations for me. Little did they know that I would prove them wrong.

Senior school brought its own traumas with the pressure of passing exams, but despite this I had now come to realise that I wanted to work with children. So armed with this desire I applied to college some distance from my home town to undertake a two-year Nursery Nursing course (NNEB). When I look back and reflect upon this, I honestly think it was the turning point for me. I moved away from home at the age of 16 and made a new start. The college tutors and the new friends I made had no preconceived ideas about me or my lack of academic skills. So I embraced every aspect of the NNEB course and passed with flying colours. At this point, as a nursery nurse, I did not know that I would move into nursing and I certainly did not have long enough vision to see that I would move into education.

I moved to London as a private nanny and enjoyed all that the capital city had to offer. A college friend of mine always wanted to be a nurse and kept badgering me to apply with her. So I applied to do what was then the SRN (State Registered Nursing). My friend met a boy, fell in love, and never became a nurse, which today I think she still regrets!

Getting into nursing for me was not easy as my school qualifications were sadly lacking, and at interviews I can remember the nurse tutors saying to me 'If you are serious about a nursing career we suggest you go back to college and get some more qualifications.' This was very traumatic but thankfully one of the schools of nursing gave me a chance. They invited me to take what was then the GNC (General Nursing Council) entrance exam. (The GNC was the equivalent of today's NMC.) I thought I am sunk, as the exam was an IQ test, which was clearly not going to be my forte! To my complete surprise (and I must say to the surprise of my family) I passed the exam and was offered a place on the nurse training course. Once again I passed first time and became a state registered nurse.

Since then I have never looked back. I followed my dream of working with children by completing my sick children's nurse training. I am a true reflection of a lifelong learner – I subsequently passed a master's degree, gained a postgraduate diploma in education, published articles and presented at conferences on a local, national and international basis.

My experience as a Senior Lecturer and Admissions Tutor has been the catalyst for this book. Answering daily emails and telephone calls from prospective students made me realise that there was a gap in the market for a text such as this.

During my incredible nursing career I have embraced every opportunity that presented itself and every new job has expanded my desire to learn more and share what I have learnt. This is probably what led me into education, as I saw the opportunity of working with student nurses to encourage them to harness their potential and be the best they can.

I think what I am really trying to say here is that if you truly have passions about becoming a nurse, follow your dreams but make absolutely sure that you know what you are embarking on. This book has been written with the help of my expert colleagues to assist you in making your decisions about embarking on a nursing career. The application process can be confusing for all, including for those nurses who are contemplating returning to nursing practice. It is very much hoped that this book will help you to navigate your way into nursing and provide an insight into what to expect from your nurse training, and it offers some heartfelt testimonials from student nurses.

Finally I want to wish you well in whatever area of nursing you find yourself, and hope that you have an incredible career voyage. Don't forget there is a world of nursing out there, and if I can do it with my rocky academic start then so can you. All you have to do is be committed and motivated – and the rest will follow.

Acknowledgements

I would like to say a huge thank you to all my expert colleagues from both the academic and clinical environments who have helped me to complete this book. Without their contributions this book would have remained an embryonic idea. I would also like to apologise to them for my doggedness in chasing deadlines and hope that they can forgive me.

I would also like to express my gratitude to the student nurses who contributed to this book, providing honest and heartfelt testimonials.

Lastly I would like to say a big thank you to Zophia who stepped into the breach and provided her artistic skills through the provision of the cartoons.

Abbreviations

APEL	Accreditation of prior and experiential learning
BOSS	Bursary online support system
C&YP	Children and young people
CAMHS	Child and adolescent mental health services
CNM	Certified nurse midwife
CNS	Clinical nurse specialist
CPD	Continuous professional development
CPPD	Continuous personal and professional development
DBS	Disclosure and Barring Service
DCMH	Defence Centre for Mental Health
DH	Department of Health
DMS	Defence Medical Services
DNF	Defence Nursing Forum
DSA	Disabled Students' Allowance
GMC	General Medical Council
GNC	General Nursing Council
GP	General Practitioner
HCA	Health care assistant
HCPC	Health & Care Professions Council
HE	Higher education
HEE	Health Education England
HEI	Higher education institution
IELTS	International English language testing system
IQ	Intelligence quotient
LETBs	Local education training boards
MDHUs	Ministry of Defence hospital units
MDT	Multi-disciplinary team
MH	Mental health
MHA	Mental Health Act
MoD	Ministry of Defence
NARIC	National Academic Recognition Information Centre
NCB	Non-credit bearing
NHS	National Health Service
NMC	Nursing and Midwifery Council
NP	Nurse practitioner

NSS	National student survey
OSCEs	Objective structured clinical examinations
PICU	Paediatric intensive care unit
PMLD	Profound multiple learning disabilities
Prep	Post-registration education and practice
RCDM	Royal Centre for Defence Medicine
RCN	Royal College of Nursing
RGN	Registered general nurse
RMN	Registered mental nurse
RN	Registered nurse
RNT	Registered nurse tutor
TOEFL	Test of English as a foreign language
UCAS	Universities & Colleges Admissions Service
WBL	Work-based learning

Contributors

Lisa Abbott RN (Child), BSc (Hons), MA (Education) undertook her Children's Nurse training in Manchester, and upon qualifying she moved back to the West Midlands to begin her nursing career in Paediatric Intensive Care (PICU). Lisa combined her passion for intensive care nursing with travelling, and nursed her way around Australia. On her return Lisa undertook the role of Lecturer Practitioner supporting students during their placements on PICU.

Now as a Senior Lecturer at Birmingham City University, Lisa has a keen interest in enhancing students' employability and ensuring they successfully undergo the transition from student nurse to registered nurse.

Tim Badger RN (Adult), MSc, BSc (Hons) is Programme Director, School of Nursing, Midwifery and Social Work Professions, Birmingham City University. Tim trained as a State Registered Nurse in Birmingham and qualified in 1980. He then worked for several years in acute medical wards and cardiac units in both Birmingham and Leicester. Whilst working as a charge nurse in coronary care he developed his interest in teaching, which encouraged him to develop his academic skills with a Diploma in Nursing from the University of London and an education degree from Wolverhampton.

Working at an HEI since 1995, Tim has taught nursing students at all stages of their training and is currently programme director for Return to Nursing.

Stefan Cash MA Ed, PG Cert. (Oxon), PG Cert. Res., BA (Hons), RN (Child), RNT, QN, FHEA has held senior nursing positions within both the hospital and community settings, as well as in Directorate Management and Higher Education. Stefan's clinical and academic speciality lies in emergency paediatrics and Child Health. In 2012 Stefan was awarded the prestigious Queen's Nurse Title for his commitment to patient values and improving practice. Stefan currently works as a Senior Lecturer at Birmingham City University.

Ann-Marie Dodson RN (Adult), BSc, PG Cert. Ed. has had a long and varied career in nursing since joining the NHS in 1977 as a nursing auxiliary whilst at university and needing a summer job. She has never looked back and is still passionate about caring for patients and empowering students and staff to develop professionally and personally.

She has experience in intensive care, transplantation, teaching, counselling, management and student nurse admissions. Whilst working in an HEI she has developed a keen interest in employability and is currently developing overseas opportunities for student nurses and other allied health professionals to explore the Himalayas and work with street children in Kathmandu, Nepal. Ann-Marie currently works as a Senior Lecturer at Birmingham City University.

Carol Doyle RN (Adult), RN (Child), Cert. Ed (FE), BSc, MA is Head of the School of Nursing, Midwifery and Social Work Professions at Birmingham City University. She has responsibility for practice placements, skills and simulation, physiology and professional development within the Faculty of Health. Carol qualified as a nurse at East Birmingham Hospital, specialising in thoracic surgical nursing and as a sick children's nurse at Great Ormond Street Hospital. Her interest in teaching evolved from her role as a mentor with students in practice. She has been involved in nurse education since 1987 in various posts, including being a lecturer/practitioner, which has led to a special interest in all elements of practice competency and its assessment, plus skills development through simulation.

Jon Harrison RN (Child), BNurs. (Hons), PG Cert., PG Dip., MA (Education). In 2001 Jon qualified as a Children's Nurse after completing his degree at the University of Birmingham. Jon has experience in neonatal intensive care, accident and emergency and in general medical and surgical care for children and young people. Prior to becoming a Senior Lecturer at Birmingham City University, Jon enjoyed a year working as a Clinical Teacher where he was actively involved in supporting nursing students with their practice learning experience.

Catharine Jenkins RMN, Diploma in Community Mental Health Nursing, BA (Hons), MSc, Cert. Ed and PG Dip Education, PG Cert. Training in Dementia Care. Working as a Senior Lecturer at Birmingham City University, Catharine teaches at all levels on mental health, specialising in the mental health of older people. She has a particular interest in dementia care and is currently involved in research on the competencies required by specialist practitioners working in the dementia care field.

She is also particularly interested in creative approaches to active learning for nurse education. Prior to becoming a nurse educator, Catharine worked for many years as a Community Mental Health Nurse and team leader of an outreach team. At present she also works as a volunteer for BUDS (Better Understanding of Dementia in Sandwell).

Ruth Lawton BA (Hons), Dip CG, PG Cert., FSEDA, FHEA is University Learning and Teaching Fellow for Employability at Birmingham City University and works in the Centre for Enhancement of Learning & Teaching. Ruth is a trained and experienced careers adviser who now works with individual academic and student support staff and course teams as they embed employability in their practice. She still works with students and graduates, including using her coaching qualification and experience. Ruth's interests are in the practical application of employability – equipping people to be successful in their life and career.

Judy Lewis-Basson RN (Adult), RNT, BSc (Hons) Nursing Studies, MA (Education), Fellow of the Higher Education Academy. Working as a Senior Lecturer at Birmingham City University, Judy co-ordinates a nursing module within the BSc nursing programme, Health in Society. Her particular area of expertise is pain management, and she facilitates sessions on this topic across the three years of the nursing programme and continues to work in clinical practice as part of a pain management team at a local hospital trust. Her other areas of interest include trauma and orthopaedic nursing and student support in clinical practice, working in partnership with a local trust's visiting students and mentors supporting and enhancing learning experiences for students.

Marie O'Boyle-Duggan RN (Learning Disability), MA Education. Marie has 32 years' experience working in a wide range of services for people with learning disabilities (including autistic spectrum conditions and challenging needs) as a residential care manager, community nurse, and behaviour specialist nurse. She is currently a Senior Lecturer in nursing at Birmingham City University and has trained in Applied Behaviour Analysis in the use of positive behaviour support. She also specialises in sexuality and sexual health of people with learning disabilities.

Her research MA in Education involved using actors to portray patients with severe learning disabilities to act out/simulate clinical scenarios with health students to explore reasonable adjustments and attitudes towards patients with learning disabilities in mainstream healthcare settings.

Trevor Parker MSc, BSc (Hons) Health Studies, RN (Adult) qualified as an enrolled nurse whilst serving in the Army, converting this status to an RGN qualification at Dartford and Gravesham in the 1980s. He has gained a range of clinical/educational experience and knowledge working for a number of different organisations and had experience in theatres, elderly care, acute care, and renal and respiratory medicine before moving into professional development.

As Practice Education Lead, Trevor is passionate about ensuring students are well prepared to become excellent parts of the future workforce. He works with practice mentors and assessors to ensure they act as effective role models, enthusiastic teachers and rigorous gatekeepers to the caring professions.

Debbie Pittaway RN (Adult), BSc (Hons), MSc spent her career in the perioperative environment, developing a keen interest in pain management. For the last 25 years she has worked in education, delivering pre- and post-qualification programmes for nurses and allied health professionals. She has a passion for travel and seeking new experiences. Five years ago she realised this dream, not only to travel but live and work in Australia. Upon returning to the UK, Debbie decided to seek a new challenge. She now works as a freelance educational consultant for local Trusts and higher education institutions.

Cathy Poole RN (Adult), RN (Child), MSc Public Sector Management, PG Dip Education, NNEB. With over 33 years' experience in health and education Cathy has held positions in adult orthopaedics, children's nursing, nursing management, the private sector and the higher education sector. Her main area of interest is renal nursing and Cathy maintains her clinical professional development as a Bank Staff Nurse at a Children's Hospice.

Cathy is now employed as the Training and Education Manager by Fresenius Medical Care Renal Services Ltd (FMC), the world's largest provider of dialysis products and dialysis care. She maintains her interest in pre-registration student nurse training as an external examiner for the BSc Nursing Programme at the University of Brighton. Additionally she works actively with other higher education institutions across the UK establishing clinical nursing placements within the FMC satellite haemodialysis units for student nurses undertaking their adult nurse training. Cathy also promotes access to learning beyond registration for the registered nurses employed by FMC in the UK and Ireland.

Fiona Rich RN (Learning Disability), DPSN, BSc (Hons) Nursing, MSc Advanced Nursing Practice, Diploma in Epilepsy Care, Cert. Ed (HE) qualified as a learning disability nurse in 1986 but has also developed a keen interest in epilepsy care. She became a Senior Lecturer in Learning Disability Nursing in 1995 and has been involved in both pre- and post-qualification nurse education in a number of roles, including Pathway Leader, Field Leader, Deputy Programme Director and Admissions Tutor at Birmingham City University.

Fiona is also involved in developing interactive virtual learning environments to educate both pre- and post-qualified nurses in the complex needs of people with learning disabilities and has travelled throughout Europe to showcase these virtual teaching tools.

Bethann Siviter Dip HE Nsg BSc (Hons) SPDN District Nurse is a UK Registered Nurse and nursing author who is best known as the author of *The Student Nurse Handbook*. Her passion for nursing and experiences as a disabled person are often explored in both her writing and speaking. When she first moved to the UK, delays in translating her nursing qualification resulted in her becoming a nursing student. She became a member of the RCN's Student Association, then its chair, and her advocacy and passion for UK nurse education was born. After contributing to the RCN's vision for Nurse Education, she participated in the Nursing and Midwifery Council's work to redevelop pre-registration nursing standards, ensuring recognition and support for disabled students as well as supporting compassionate, person-focused nursing care. As a Consultant Nurse, CQC Specialist Advisor and independent nursing consultant, she has continued to promote and support nursing care delivered with skill, knowledge and genuine caring.

Suzan Smallman RSCN, RGN, RNT, LLB Hons, MSc, NDN Cert. has had a varied and stimulating career. Since completing her training as a nurse in 1978, she has had the opportunity to work at both local and national level and in clinical practice, management and education. Her primary interest is in quality of care and patient standards and this has been demonstrated in her involvement in developing clinical standards, policy and educational audit.

She is presently working as an independent consultant in healthcare and maintains her clinical skills through occasional work at a children's hospice.

Anthony Tuckett RN, MA (Research), PhD trained at the Princess Alexandra Hospital in Brisbane. He back-packed through Europe, where he also cared for the elderly in their homes, and then went overland from Nairobi to Harare.

Anthony is Courses Coodinator, Master of Nursing (Aged Care Management) for the School of Nursing, Midwifery and Social Work at the University of Queensland, and has 20-plus years' experience in the tertiary education of and curriculum development for nurses. He conducts research in residential aged care, nursing workforce/workplace, and dabbles in applied ethics.

Kate Wadley MA(Ed), PGCE, BSc (Hons), Community health studies, DPSN, RGN qualified as an enrolled nurse in 1980 in Birmingham. She then completed a district enrolled nurse course and worked in Balsall Heath, an inner city area of Birmingham. After completing a specialist practitioner degree she became a district nurse team leader in a similar area. Kate was always interested in nurse education and in 2000 was one of the first clinical placement co-ordinators employed following the Peach Report (1999).

The role has changed over the years but its main aim is to ensure that student healthcare professionals are working in a clinical environment that is conducive to learning.

Tony Whittle RN (Adult), MSc Advanced Practice, BSc (Hons) Education Studies, DPSN is currently the Director of CPD at the Faculty of Health, Education and Life Sciences, Birmingham City University. Since becoming a qualified tutor in 1982, he has worked primarily with the post registration field of nurse and clinical education.

As Director Tony is involved in all aspects of CPD delivery from the faculty and a particular interest at present is the expansion and availability of work-based learning within the NHS and beyond. His teaching interests are currently in health assessment and within individual independent-based learning, enabling practitioners to study topics allied to their personal and professional development.

Fang Yu RN, PhD, GNP-BC was born and raised in mainland China. She entered nursing serendipitously – admitted by Peking University School of Nursing instead of Medicine. After practising nursing for two years after graduation, Fang went to the US and obtained her Master's as a Gerontological Nurse Practitioner and her PhD from the University of Pennsylvania.

After completing a postdoctoral fellowship, Fang began her faculty position and is currently a tenured Associate Professor at the University of Minnesota School of Nursing. She is a well-recognised researcher, teacher, and mentor in nursing, gerontology and dementia.

Introduction

Is this book for me?

Well, if you are considering joining the nursing profession, or returning to nursing practice then the answer is 'Yes'. This book has been written with you in mind, and aims to steer you through what can, on the face of it, be a complicated process. For those of you who are just starting to think about applying to undertake your nurse training this book has been structured in such a way that it will provide you with vital information to help you make your decisions about which field of nursing to choose, how to navigate UCAS and be successful in your nursing application – and in your ongoing nursing career.

How the book is organised

Part 1 is dedicated to providing you with an understanding of nursing. It introduces the definition of nursing, incorporating an overview of the history of nursing in order to afford some key background to this established career choice. Also included is an introduction to the role played by men in nursing and the misconceptions about nursing.

Part 2 provides an insight into the uniqueness of the four fields of nursing (adult, child, mental health, learning disabilities) in order to assist you in making your final choice. This will include what you can expect to learn, the teaching and learning strategies adopted, the methods of assessment of learning, and where you will gain clinical nursing skills. Also included is a description of defence nursing, providing information for applicants not only embarking on a career in nursing but also a military career.

Part 3 focuses on the process of applying for nursing courses at higher education institutions through the Universities & Colleges Admissions Service (UCAS). Detail is provided concerning the UCAS cycles, with information relating to the tariff system and tracking process. This section also aims to uncover the skills and qualities required to become a nurse, and draws upon the professional regulations stipulated by the NMC. In addition, it provides key information and advice for nurses who are considering a return to nursing programme.

Part 4 serves to outline the support that students can expect during their nurse training programme from an academic and clinical standpoint, which will also include the potential for reasonable adjustments for students with disabilities. It also places focus on the potential stresses of being a student nurse and the strategies which can be adopted to deal with these stresses.

Part 5 concentrates on what to expect when you complete your nurse training programme. There are sections on employability skills, securing your first job, nursing around the globe and the notion of embarking on a journey of lifelong learning.

In summary, the logical format of this book is contextualised in Figure 0.1. It is not our intention that this book be read from cover to cover but is viewed more as a resource to be dipped in and out of, depending on which point of your nursing career you are at.

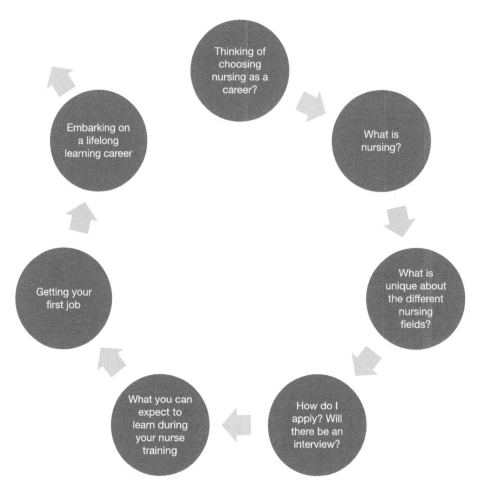

Figure 0.1 The cyclical vision for the book

Part 1

Understanding nursing

Chapter 1

Defining nursing

Ann-Marie Dodson

I remember that the reaction when we had to study Nursing History in our training was one of groans and horror. My peers would say 'Why can't we spend more time learning about physiology? That's much more useful to patient care.' I could appreciate this viewpoint to some extent. I still hear this comment today from some students and of course we all as individuals have our own interests and preferences – that is what makes people so interesting and individual. Now, having been a nurse and teacher for many years (and latterly an Admissions Tutor) I have come to appreciate, that for many reasons, it is important to have some understanding of what a healthcare profession is, how it has developed and what influences exist that will develop it further to shape the National Health Service (NHS) of the future and meet the needs of patients. So, as well as having some knowledge of nursing history, misconceptions about nursing and understanding what nursing is, it is important to understand the educational, sociological and political influences that have an interplay on the profession.

One moment in my career development where this knowledge really helped me was when I had a panel interview for my first senior post as a sister. I was able to talk about the development of the NHS and its management structures. I was able to explain how the NHS had evolved. How various reorganisations had impacted on service delivery and patient care, how things would develop in the future, and how I would develop the sister's nursing post. I got the job and the feedback was about how impressed the panel were by my knowledge. That was an important reflective or learning moment for me, as it was the moment I was fully aware that to be effective in a system you need to know how it has developed, where you fit into it and how you can influence it. This is why politicians and military leaders often have an interest in history. By learning about the lessons from the past we can influence things in the future. As well as historical factors there are also the sociological and political influences that nurses must be aware of.

The following sections outline how nursing has developed as a profession in the UK, particularly in England. This seemingly narrow and parochial approach is necessary as, although there are similarities with other countries, there are also differences too. For example, although nursing in English-speaking countries such as the US and Australia is extremely similar, there can be distinct differences too in what nurses do and how they are prepared educationally. An example of this was when I spent some time in an American intensive care unit. In Britain, I would decide when I wanted to take a blood sample to check the patient's oxygen levels and alter the ventilator accordingly. I would not need to consult a doctor unless I had concerns, or needed them to do a review and change the treatment plan. The patients were sedated to make the experience less distressing for them. I had an element of autonomy.

In the US I had to get a 'Doctor's order' to be able to take the blood sample, and the ventilator would then be altered by a Respiratory Technician. The patient was restrained by leather straps as they were not sedated. Yet, the nurses by comparison were very highly educated to degree, Master's and doctorate level, which we were not at that time, and they were able to clinically assess a patient – which again we did not do.

My experiences lately of travelling in parts of China, India and Nepal have outlined other differences whereby, in some provinces, the role of the nurse is to carry out some of the treatments prescribed by the doctor (what we used to describe historically as the 'doctor's hand-maiden role') and it is the family who stay in the hospital and deliver what we consider to be the nursing care; so they wash, feed and generally meet the care needs of their loved one. In some of these cultures there are not usually any male nurses (see Chapter 2 for more information on men in nursing). Clearly, these differences in nursing across the world develop due to cultural, educational and socio-economic and political factors.

So what is nursing? The next section will set out some ideas to help you define what *you* think nursing is.

As an Admissions Tutor, part of my role is to ascertain if prospective candidates have the necessary qualities and attributes to be a nurse, as well as meeting the required educational qualifications. The interviewing teams will try to draw out what the candidate understands to be the role of the nurse and what nursing is. This is important for two reasons. First, we want to ensure that the candidate has undertaken some research and is making an informed choice for the right reasons. Further information relating to this is discussed in depth in Part 3 'How to become a nurse'. Nursing is hard physical work and can be psychologically demanding, involving long and unsocial hours. Choosing nursing needs to be an appropriate choice for you, but also for the patients who you will be looking after.

Secondly, as each university place carries an NHS bursary it is important that there is a strong likelihood that you will be able to cope with the academic level of the training, successfully complete the clinical placements, and qualify as a Registered Nurse. Some candidates are extremely well prepared and have an excellent understanding of what nursing 'is' and what nurses 'do'. However some do not. This chapter may help give you some insight into these aspects and help you prepare more effectively.

I had always wanted to be a nurse since the age of three or four. This surely wasn't because I knew what nursing was. As I grew older this desire did not diminish. I liked looking after people, being helpful, easing discomfort and problem solving. I was the one that friends and peers came to if they needed to discuss a problem. I dealt with accidents from a young age and was calm in a crisis. I truly believe that if you can find the match between your personality and the job, then you too will have a lifetime of happiness and satisfaction, and be good at what you do.

However, neither my parents nor my school wanted me to pursue my dream, as nursing was considered a waste of a good education and was just a job or an occupation – and certainly not a profession. Some of these preconceptions and myths will be explored later.

What is nursing?

A first-year nursing student said to me recently that nursing 'was about putting the patient first and going the extra mile'. I think about it being a 'social interaction' whereby I can do

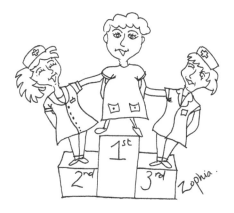

something for someone else which they cannot do themselves. Or I can help them find new ways of doing something, in the case of disability or poor health. Increasingly, nursing is about empowering individuals to be able to live healthily and access health services.

'Nursing' and 'caring' are synonymous but caring is not necessarily unique to nursing, as doctors and radiographers feel they are caring and deliver care. Indeed, there has been media criticism that many nurses are 'uncaring', and there is debate about how and if this attribute or quality can be taught.

Caring is a fundamental human attribute that is necessary for human growth, development and, most importantly, survival. Brown *et al.* (1992: 31) said that 'a capacity for caring is part of human nature'. As a nurse, this involves the ability to understand some of the situation the other person is in and to be able to feel for that other person. Psychologists and counsellors describe this as *empathy*. Like mastering any other skill, it needs to be worked at, understood, refined and made sense of. The relationship of caring to nursing needs to be understood. The nurse could be described as a 'professional carer' and nursing as the professionalisation of caring. Leninger, an influential American nurse theorist, believes that caring is 'the central and unifying domain for the body of knowledge practices in Nursing' (1981: 3).

Nursing is an 'art' and 'science'. The 'art' is a collection of the soft caring and communication skills. The 'science' is all the underpinning theoretical knowledge from the sciences, such as physiology and pharmacology. The good nurse will be able to balance the science and the art so that care given is both competent and effective and of a quality recognised by both patients and professionals. The good nurse will be altering these aspects according to the situation and the patient being nursed.

What do academics say that nursing is? How is it defined?

Henderson (1966) provided a classic and seminal definition of nursing which focuses on the unique function of the nurse in terms of assisting individuals whether sick or well to be able to perform a defined list of activities which contribute to health or recovery or indeed to a peaceful death. Henderson further explains that nurses play a role in helping individuals to gain independence as rapidly as possible.

This definition acknowledges implicitly that life is a continuum from birth to death and implies that, as nurses, we can't always make things better and have happy endings, but what we can do is our best for the patient (and their family or loved ones) in every situation.

The Royal College of Nursing appears to have built on Henderson's 1966 definition, by defining nursing as:

> the use of clinical judgement in the provision of care to enable people to improve, maintain or recover health, to cope with health problems, and to achieve the best possible quality of life, whatever their disease or disability, until death.
>
> (RCN 2003: 3)

The regulatory body, the Nursing and Midwifery Council (NMC), that protects the public and sets the standards for pre-registration Nursing and Midwifery programmes also utilised the RCN (2003) definition. In the NMC standards for pre-registration programmes it states that the nurse should be:

> a safe, caring, and competent decision maker, willing to accept personal and professional accountability for his/her actions and continuous learning.
>
> (NMC 2010: 11)

Recently, the Chief Nursing Officer for England, Jane Cummings (DH 2012a), introduced the concept of the 6 C's to restore publicly the notion of compassion and caring, which nurses have been accused of losing.

You can see from the various definitions that nursing is made up of many roles, attributes, attitudes and skills. There are currently four fields of nursing (adult, child, mental health, and learning disability) at pre-registration level, which will be discussed in Part 2 of this book. After qualifying, nurses will go and study further and perhaps specialise (see Part 5). There are so many different types of nurses – School Nurses, Diabetic Specialist Nurses, and Intensive Care Nurses, for example. What unites them is their ability to communicate and form relationships with patients, in order to assess, plan, and deliver and evaluate care. They need to be able to draw on a wide knowledge base, teach, promote health, and make decisions. They need to be able to problem solve, delegate,

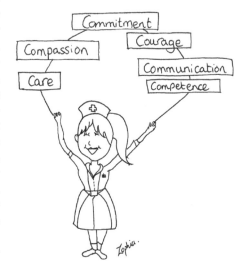

supervise and manage care. The current NMC (2010) standards for pre-registration nursing education document has outlined various professional and clinical competencies which are gathered into four domains of practice:

- Professional values
- Communications and interpersonal skills
- Nursing practice and decision making
- Leadership, management and team working.

Now that there has been some exploration of what caring and nursing are in general terms, the following section gives some context to the history and development of nursing.

Overview of the history of nursing

Caring, healing and nursing (derived from the Latin for 'nourishing') are all intertwined historically. There is not always a consensus in the literature. For instance, the Feminist writers feel that history is written from a male paternalistic perspective (Baly 1995).

Additionally, not until recent times has Mary Seacole, a Black Jamaican nurse, been recognised for her contribution to nursing, which equals that of Florence Nightingale.

It is not possible to cover every aspect of the historical evolution of nursing as we would need to cover thousands of years of development across the world. Therefore, the main points will be covered to give a broad overview.

Where have we come from as a profession?

Nursing has been struggling to be viewed as a true profession, partly because traditionally nurses have not possessed a unique knowledge base or full autonomy. Doctors on the other hand diagnose and prescribe medications and treatments. However this position is changing, and the development of nurses' roles are such that Donahue (1996: 2) said that 'Nursing has been called the oldest of the arts and the youngest of the professions.'

Mothering and nursing are synonymous and instinctual, in women particularly (although this does not mean that men cannot be caring), and untrained 'nurses' are as old as the human race. Initially, it was predominantly about caring for infants and being home based. It was a sensible division of labour, as the men were out hunting and defending the property, whilst the women were bringing up the children. This is still the pattern in many more rural economies in the world.

There was a time when we were much closer to nature, and herbs, leaves and seeds were used as magical cures. As early as 20,000 BC there were depictions in caves of Shamanistic activities (Keegan 1988). At one time a mother would pass down such knowledge of healing and herbs to her daughters. Later men got involved in this esoteric knowledge and skill as bone-setters, medicine men, witch doctors or Shamans. This art of healing set them aside from the tribe and there was the development of this medicine, not just for healing and good, but also for bad, as 'occult' medicine.

By 500 BC in Greece, Hippocrates had developed a scientific medicine through rationality and observation. Healing and caring had moved out of the home and become a broader function. The Greeks and Romans were influential in the development of medicine and nursing. Nursing pre-dated medicine, but the two became interwoven as time elapsed. Around 100 BC the Romans constructed 'valetudinarias' which were buildings designed to care for sick gladiators, soldiers and slaves, and thus military nursing evolved. During the Crusades, the Knights Hospitallers (Knights of St John) were a military nursing order. Military nursing is not a new phenomenon and has long informed civilian practice. (For further information on this aspect of nursing, see Chapter 4.)

Caring became a more organised activity in communities linked to monasticism. The monks nursed the men in male wards, and women were nursed separately by nuns. Later these communities moved into closed orders as the deacons and deaconesses wanted to be removed from materialism – and secular care/medicine was gone.

As trades evolved, with a move away from an agrarian society, guilds were formed. Barbers and surgeons became affiliated together because of the commonality of bleeding – as did apothecaries and physicians because of the affiliation of chemicals.

In the sixteenth century, the split from the Roman Catholic Church caused the destruction and dissolution of monasteries. Although there were still religious nursing orders being founded, such as the French order of Vincent de Paul, the growth of more secular nursing orders was seen. These had no specific religious ties but continued to use the term Nursing 'Sister', thus maintaining strong religious connotations.

Ultimately, it was felt that communities should pay for and look after the sick and needy of their own parish. In 1601 the Elizabethan Poor Law was introduced. Some say this was the 'dark period of nursing'. Poor Law hospitals were created and most of the care was delivered by the inmates.

In 1834, the Poor Law Amendment Act was passed. The Poor Law hospitals, paid for by the parish rate, became places to be dreaded, like the 'workhouses'. At the same time, however, voluntary hospitals were being created from contributions from wealthy patrons and doctors. They were selective as to who was admitted – for instance children and people with infectious diseases were excluded. These institutions became teaching establishments and, later, medical schools. They attracted middle-class women who wanted financial security and greater occupational status than the Poor Law Nurses, who were seen as more like domestic servants, often of a disreputable nature. Nursing in voluntary hospitals was more than domestic duty and some training was given by surgeons and physicians.

Specialisms began to develop, as the mentally ill ('lunatics'), the feeble minded and those with infectious diseases were located outside the city boundaries to protect the public. When the Mental Deficiency Act was introduced in 1913, the mentally ill and the mentally handicapped (those with learning disabilities) were separated. The staff who worked in the asylums were the first to have a training register from 1890. This work was mainly carried out by men, because it involved violent patients and restraint with a penal aspect. For further information on mental health and learning disability nursing, see Part 2, where you will discover the uniqueness of these nursing fields.

So nursing had moved from caring for infants to caring for the sick in the eighteenth century. Although there were the 'Sarah Gamp' gin wife characters described by Dickens and depicted in Hogarth's drawings, in the nineteenth century nursing did become a more organised activity under the direction of a physician. Nurses who were affiliated to a religious order were altruistic – it was a life of service and self-sacrifice.

After a whistle stop tour of the development of nursing from ancient times through the Middle Ages we reach the huge influences of Elizabeth Fry, Florence Nightingale, Bedford Fenwick and Mary Seacole. This is the advent of what we recognise as 'modern nursing'.

Modern nursing

Elizabeth Fry (1780–1845) was a prison visitor and prototype social worker. Although she was not a nurse she was influential in her work in advocating social reform and recognising inequalities in health.

Florence Nightingale (1820–1910) was an educated upper-class woman who brought respectability to nursing through her work with the military in Turkey during the Crimean War in the 1850s. Mary Seacole (1805–1881), although contributing significantly in the Crimea and subsequently to raise the profile and influence of nursing, has only been recognised fully in recent times, maybe because of her mixed race and lower social status. Whatever the politics and reality of history, Nightingale's contribution is truly amazing, especially as she was in ill health for much of her life after the Crimean War. Apart from her seminal book, *Notes on Nursing*, published in 1860, she contributed to infection control, statistics, nursing theory (with knowledge of the environment and nutrition) and the organisation and management of care (Hegge 2011).

Mrs (Ethel) Bedford Fenwick (1857–1947) had much in common with Nightingale, as they each set up their own nurse training schools (Nightingale at St Thomas' and Bedford

Fenwick at St Bartholomew's). But they were also adversaries when it came to the notion of state registration of nurses. Bedford Fenwick led the middle-class lobby for registration which was based in the voluntary hospitals. Nightingale was against registration and felt that it was more important to recruit the right type or character of probationer. In 1897 the campaign began, culminating in the Nurses Registration Act 1919, and Ethel Bedford Fenwick appeared as 'Nurse No. 1' when the register opened in 1923.

The International Council of Nurses was formed in 1899. At this time, American nurses were forging ahead in terms of their development and education – perhaps because they were not entrenched in the same class and power systems.

After the Second World War a second level of registration had to be created, which was meant to be a 'roll' rather than register to acknowledge the work of stretcher bearers and field orderlies. This led later to a new 'Enrolled Nurse' status following a shorter two-year training with more bedside experience.

It wasn't until 1989 that nurses were finally in control of their own profession with the formation of the United Kingdom Central Council for Nursing and Midwifery (UKCC) which brought nine regulatory bodies under one organisation (and closing the register for infectious disease nursing for instance). This body existed until 2001 with the advent of the current Nursing and Midwifery Council.

With the introduction of the UKCC came the abolition of the apprenticeship-style training and the final state examination. 'Project 2000', a totally new curriculum and style of training and education, saw the relocation of Schools of Nursing based on hospital sites to universities. Students became supernumerary to the NHS workforce and bursaried. A third of the curriculum was theory and the remainder practice, with an 18-month common foundation programme and an academic qualification, as well as registration at the end. However, after criticism that these nurses were felt to be inferior to those trained under the apprenticeship system another new curriculum was developed, 'Making a difference' (DH 1999). This incorporated more skills, which many felt were missing from Project 2000. The Project 2000 nurses were viewed with scepticism as they were felt to be too academic and not fit for purpose at the point of qualification. Therefore, the new revised curriculum focused on the notion of 'fitness to practice'. It changed the theory/practice split to 50/50. More skills were incorporated with a period of consolidation prior to qualification. The common foundation element was reduced to one year, with a two-year branch-specific component. This curriculum has been re-crafted in the 2010 NMC standards with the branch of nursing being replaced by fields of nursing and no common foundation. The programme is now all degree level. This is a major and fundamental change (although there have been nursing degrees since the 1960s in the UK). It can be argued that, by increasing the university entry criteria and making the curriculum more academic, those prospective candidates with the desired personal skills and attributes but lacking the educational qualifications will now not have the opportunity to become registered nurses. We need to counterbalance the changing needs of patients and the NHS with the education and training of nurses. Can you see repeated patterns?

Where are we currently? And where are we going?

Change started to escalate in the 1960s with the introduction of the Salmon Report (Ministry of Health 1966). Men were becoming more established in nursing, requiring some relabelling of job titles – the 'Matron' became the 'Nursing Officer', for example. However, a bigger change was when Margaret Thatcher and the Conservative Government wanted to encourage people to be less dependent on the welfare state, making people responsible for their own lives. Thus began the introduction of an industrial business method of managing health services, focused on efficiency and effectiveness (Griffiths 1983). With the growing public and media perception that healthcare quality was diminishing in recent times, the concept of the 'Modern matron' was introduced (Secretary of State 2000).

The pace of change and its impact continues to escalate. It seems that politicians now realise that healthcare costs are exponential, and that the country cannot sustain them – or the NHS in the current format. So, where are we going?

In recent times, the government, the media and the public have been quite critical of poor nursing practices and the attitudes of some nurses, which has had a disproportionate negative influence. A lot of questioning has arisen about the appropriateness of the current nurse training. There have been accusations that nurses today are less caring and compassionate, for instance. The RCN (2012) are so concerned about this critique and undermining of the nursing position, particularly around the training and education of nursing students, that they have asked a peer, Lord Willis (2012), to form an Independent Commission to carry out an inquiry to examine the future of nurse education. It appears that many nurses are very disgruntled with the nursing regulatory body (NMC). It has been under much scrutiny and criticism because of a backlog of disciplinary hearings and allegations of poor management. This process may lead to nursing losing its own regulatory body, and being subsumed under the Health Care Professions Council (HCPC) with other allied health professionals, such as physiotherapists and dieticians. The General Medical Council (GMC), the doctors' regulatory body, has also been under this scrutiny and may suffer the same fate, which has the potential to reduce doctor/nurse autonomy and power.

Of course, there are good and bad in every profession, and it seems that the few bad spoil it for the many. Some of the criticisms of poor care are levelled at 'nurses', but I suspect that some of the culprits of poor care are unregistered staff (although ultimately a registered nurse will be responsible for overseeing the care). It is often difficult for patients and their families to differentiate between the various members of the nursing teams and some NHS Trusts are trying to deal with this. Having nurses trained at diploma and degree level has also led to some confusion. However, it is no different in the US where there are associate, bachelor, masters and doctoral level nurses, who all have different role functions.

As the NHS has been constantly reorganised since its inception and the nature and pace of change is escalating, especially in these times of austerity, acute services are being contracted. The number of trained nurses is also dropping so that their skill mix and workload is changing, and quality of care will be impacted at times. However even this is under review, with the drive to determining minimum staffing levels as a result of the Mid Staffordshire NHS Trust scandal.

The decision to move nursing from Colleges of Nursing which were generally based on hospital sites into universities heralded big changes, as the partnerships between the clinical area and the university needed to be worked at. These partnerships become disjointed, and some ownership of the curriculum appears to have been lost.

The final change for the moment has been the decision for nursing to become an all graduate profession. This will bring it in line with all the others such as physiotherapy and radiography. Already a drop in the number of nursing students has occurred, especially as the Diploma course in Nursing has now all but finished. These graduates will be supported by a growing number of support workers such as Health Care Assistants. This has already been happening as nurses take on what were previously doctors' roles such as assessment, prescribing and running their own clinics as Nurse Practitioners and Specialist Nurses.

The nurse of the future will need to be highly educated and articulate, with an ability to lead and transform services to meet the changing needs of society and the profession. The patterns of disease are changing. Many diseases are self-inflicted and lifestyle-related such as obesity, cardio-vascular disease, diabetes and abuse of alcohol and cancers. The nurse of the future will need to be an effective health promoter and motivator. With increasing longevity, more degenerative diseases will occur which will result in many more people suffering from forms of dementia. This will place an increasing burden on nursing in particular, as well as the impact socially and on the NHS.

The costs of the NHS are exponential and perhaps cannot be sustained, particularly as the economy shrinks. Many think that privatisation is the answer. The first NHS hospital to be managed by a private commercial company was Hinchingbrooke Hospital in Cambridgeshire, whose management was taken over by Circle Health in 2012. However by January 2015 Circle had decided to withdraw from the contract in the wake of an 'inadequate' assessment of care and quality by the Care Quality Commission (CQC) and financial instability. So the question now is, will there be further privatisation of NHS hospitals or will the political landscape change again and put a halt to this?

Nursing as a profession will continue to change and adapt in response to socio-economic and political influences, as it always has during its history. Nurses will always be needed, because society will always require care. This care cannot be delivered by a totally unregulated, unregistered workforce as patients expect quality care. It is clear that things can go wrong when staff are not highly trained and supervised, such as in the recent incidents in learning disabilities care homes (DH 2012b). The ongoing scientific developments and innovations in medicine mean that highly skilled nurses are required to deliver specialist care such as in transplantation and gene therapy.

The move of services into the community – although sensible to some extent to cut costs and avoid hospital-acquired infections – will have its limits, because acute hospital services will always be needed. Their training places for student nurses and other allied professionals will be vital to achieve a pertinent, balanced clinical experience. However to counterbalance these demands, technology will be harnessed more to shape services, and different methods will be used such as e-health. Health care and nursing will continue to evolve and change in these exciting times. Watch this space.

Conclusion

It is clear that nursing has undergone many changes over the centuries. Nursing remains within a dynamic arena and therefore further changes can be expected. Whatever changes evolve over the next years the fundamental principles of nursing, caring and quality of care will remain central to those changes. Nurse leaders play a pivotal role in driving the nursing agenda. They make sure that the nursing profession keeps its nursing voice and only embraces change which will have positive impacts on nurses and nursing and, most importantly, have positive impacts on patients.

References

Baly, M.E. (1995) *Nursing and Social Change*, 3rd Edn. London: Routledge.

Brown, J.M., Kitson, A.L. and McKnight, T.J. (1992) *Challenges in Caring: Explorations in Nursing and Ethics*. London: Chapman & Hall.

Department of Health (DH) (1999) *Making a Difference: Strengthening the Nursing, Midwifery and Health Visiting Contribution to Health and Healthcare*. London: DH.

Department of Health (DH) (2012a) *Compassion in Practice: Nursing, Midwifery and Care Staff: Our Vision and Strategy*. London: DH.

Department of Health (DH) (2012b) *Transforming Care: A National Response to Winterbourne View Hospital, Department of Health Review Final Report*. London: DH.

Donahue, P.M. (1996) *Nursing: The Finest Art*, 2nd Edn. London: Mosby.

Griffiths (1983) *NHS Management Inquiry*. Letter dated 6th October 1983 to the Secretary of State Norman Fowler from Roy Griffiths, Michael Betts, Jim Blyth and Sir Brian Bailey.

Hegge, M.J. (2011) The Lingering Presence of the Nightingale Legacy. *Nursing Science Quarterly* 24(2): 152–162.

Henderson, V. (1966) *The Nature of Nursing: A Definition and its Implications for Practice, Research and Education*. New York: Macmillan.

International Council for Nurses. www.icn.ch/about-icn/about-icn/ (Accessed June 5 2013).

Keegan, L. (1988) in Dossey, L., Keegan, L. and Gazzeta, C., *Holistic Nursing: A Handbook for Practice*. Gathersburg, MD: Aspen.

Leininger, M.M. (1981) Transcultural nursing: Its progress and its future. *Nursing & Health Care* 2(7): 365–371.

Ministry of Health and Scottish Home and Health Departments (1966) *Report of the Committee on Senior Nursing Staff Structure (The Salmon Report)*. London: HMSO.

Nursing and Midwifery Council (2008) *The Code: Standards of Conduct, Performance and Ethics for Nurses and Midwives*. London: Nursing and Midwifery Council.

Royal College of Nursing (2003) *Defining Nursing*. London: RCN Publishing.

Royal College of Nursing (2012) Peer Pressure. London: RCN Bulletin.

Secretary of State (2000) *The NHS Plan: A Plan for Investment, a Plan for Reform*. London: Stationery Office.

Willis (2012) *Quality with Compassion: The Future of Nursing Education (Report of the Willis Commission on Nursing Education)*. London: Royal College of Nursing.

Further reading

Basford, L. and Slevin, O. (2003) *Theory and Practice of Nursing: An Integrated Approach to Caring Practice*, 2nd Edn. Cheltenham: Nelson Thornes.

Baughan, J. and Smith, A. (2009) *Caring in Nursing Practice*. Harlow: Pearson Education.

Brooker, C. and Waugh, A. (eds) (2007) *Foundations of Nursing Practice*. London: Elsevier.

Davies, C. (1980) *Rewriting Nursing History*. London: Croom Helm.

Glasper, A., McEwing, G. and Richardson, J. (2009) *Foundation Studies for Caring*. Basingstoke: Palgrave Macmillan.

Griffith, R. and Tengnah, S. (2010) *Law and Professional Issues in Nursing*, 2nd Edn. Exeter: Learning Matters.

Kozier, B., Erb, G., Berman, B., Snyder, S., Lake, R. and Harvey, S. (2008) *Fundamentals of Nursing: Concepts, Process and Practice*. Harlow: Pearson Education.

Useful web links

Department of Health: www.dh.gov.uk
General Medical Council: www.gmc-uk.org
Government: www.direct.gov.uk
Health Care Professions Council: www.hcpc-uk.org
Nursing and Midwifery Council: www.nmc-uk.org
Royal College of Nursing: www.rcn.org.

Chapter 2

Men in nursing

Stefan Cash

The role of the male nurse has often been seen as a recent invention. This chapter, however, will provide you with a very clear insight as to exactly how long men have been involved in nursing – which may surprise you.

The blurring of social boundaries in relation to jobs, and the popularity of hospital-based TV programmes, is widely believed to be behind the trend for male nurses. However, men have always played a vital role in nursing, from 250 years BC to modern days.

Looking back

History dictates that the principles and practices of nursing are ancient. It has been suggested that the world's first nursing school was founded in India *circa* 250 BC. Interestingly, only men were considered pure enough to attend nursing school and eventually become nurses.

In the Mediterranean region in the third century, there was a group of men referred to as the Parabolani brotherhood. This brotherhood of likeminded men organised hospitals, buried the dead and delivered nursing care to the sick and dying during the great plague in Alexandria. These men were often drawn from the lower classes; they also served the dual purpose of being the attendants to local bishops. The Parabolani were sometimes used by the clergy as bodyguards and were often utilised effectively in violent clashes with their opponents (Ellis and Hartley 2012).

Early military religious and lay orders

Throughout the Middle Ages numerous male nursing orders began to emerge. Organisations such as the Alexian Brotherhood formed circa 1400 are still in existence today (Ellis & Hartley 2012).

The Congregation of Alexian Brothers is a lay Catholic order whose Brothers dedicated themselves primarily to live in the community and to participate in the ministry of healing. Some of the most famous military orders were the Knights of St John (*c*.1000), the Knights Hospitaliers (*c*.1080) and the Teutonic Knights (*c*.1100). During the crusades these orders were predominantly responsible for building and managing hospitals as well as providing nursing care to sick and injured colleagues.

Modern institutions such as St John Ambulance have their foundations in such military orders. It is widely believed that St John Ambulance originated from the Knights Hospitaller, also known as Knights of St John and Order of St John. The Hospitallers probably arose as a group of individuals associated with hospitals in Jerusalem, which were dedicated to St John the Baptist and founded around 1023 to provide care for poor, sick or injured pilgrims to the Holy Land.

Two patron saints of nursing also stem from this period. St John of God and St Camillus de Lellis both began their careers as soldiers and later dedicated their lives to nursing.

St John of God

St John of God established a dedicated circle of disciples. He organised his followers into the Order of Hospitallers, who were approved by the Holy See in 1572 as the Brothers Hospitallers of St John of God. The Brothers Hospitallers' calling was to care for the sick in countries around the world. Today there are over 1200 Brothers living and working world-wide, within 25 countries over five continents. Their mission is to meet society's needs by promoting physical, psychological, emotional and spiritual well-being.

St Camillus de Lellis

St Camillus devoted himself to caring for the sick, and became director of St Giacomo Hospital in Rome. St Camillus founded his own congregation (the Camellians), dedicated to the care of the sick. St Camillus sent members of his order to minister to wounded troops in Hungary and Croatia. Many believe this to be a description of the first field medical units. After St Camillus founded his religious order Pope Sixtus V authorised the Red Cross as a special insignia designating the special service provided by the order. The Red Cross was soon seen on many battlefields and ultimately became the insignia of organisations such as the international movement of the Red Cross and Red Crescent (Durgin & Hanan 2009). Interestingly St John of God died in 1550 the year of St Camillus' birth.

For hundreds of years nursing was largely a male-dominated occupation. In the seventeenth century there were approximately 54,000 people employed as nurses, but only a little over 1 per cent of them were women. By the turn of the eighteenth century this had grown to approximately 65,000 with a similar proportion of them being women (Traynor 2013). The advent of the wars in the nineteenth and twentieth centuries caused the nursing role to start becoming more dominated by women. Florence Nightingale has been widely cited as the catalyst in the demise of men from nursing. Historians document that Florence proposed that men were not suited to nursing and not on a par with their female counterparts (McDonald 2009).

Modern day

In the late nineteenth century nursing started to grow into a profession. With the advent of uniforms and standards of education and practice few men were found among the ranks of these 'new' nurses (Stokowski 2012). This was not entirely surprising, as nursing was one of the only professions open to women, whereas men had access to more lucrative and respected career options (Finkelman & Kenner 2010).

A common belief about nursing roles is that men prefer certain fast-paced specialty areas, such as critical care or the emergency department. Although the reasons are not entirely clear, there seems to be some truth to this belief. The top three specialties reported by men were: critical care nursing (27 per cent), emergency nursing (23 per cent), and medical/surgical nursing (20 per cent). In addition to the clinical nursing role, men reported working as middle managers (19 per cent), directors (10 per cent), educators (15 per cent) and nurse practitioners (10 per cent) (Stokowski 2012). Studies have suggested that there are some prejudices in the public attitude towards male nurses, with mental health and trauma nurses being amongst the most accepted (Mohammed 2012). The specialties reported by the fewest respondents were obstetrics/gynaecology and nursery/neonatal intensive care. Interestingly a recent study conducted by Mohammed (2012) found that male student nurses largely reported positive educational experiences. Gender was not seen as a barrier to learning and sometimes appeared to enhance learning. However, male students on gynaecological and midwifery placements felt that the constant 'polling' of patients about them gave a negative image.

Theorists such as Middleton hypothesise that

> in these times of gender equality, you might think that a profession as high profile as nursing would have a fairly balanced number of men and women. Especially when you consider that male nurses are marginally better paid and proportionally more likely to be in senior posts than their female colleagues. But despite this, the number of men entering the profession has hardly grown in recent years.
>
> (Middleton 2008)

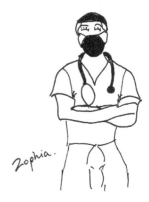

According to the most recent Nursing and Midwifery Council (NMC) figures (2008), only one in ten nurses on the register were male, a figure that has remained static for the past four years. However, this compares favourably to the United States where male nurses account for as little as 6 per cent of the register (O'Lynn 2013).

According to the NMC (2008) figures, there were 676,547 registered nurses on the register. Of the 10 per cent who were male, 53 per cent were on part 1 of the register (Adult) and 60 per cent were under the age of 40. There were only two male school nurses and 132 male midwives on the register.

Stereotyping

Nursing suffers from many female stereotypes – ranging from the doctor's handmaiden to the 'sexy' nurse. The image of men in nursing is not exempt, with many male nurses being portrayed as failed medical students or intellectually inferior. A good example would be the portrayal of Greg 'Gaylord' Focker by Ben Stiller in the films *Meet the Parents* (2000), *Meet the Fockers* (2004) and *Little Fockers* (2010). Greg's father-in-law (played by Robert de Niro) continually questions Greg's intellectual ability and manhood, with frequent suggestions that Greg should change his profession (Stokowski 2012). This view is also supported by authors such as Denny (2006) who further sums up the stereotypes of male nurses as lazy or gay. In a small study conducted by Evans (2002) on the experience of men in nursing, touch was identified as a central practice in nursing, yet problematic for male nurses. Evans suggests that male nurses feared that touching patients may be misinterpreted and that they may be accused of inappropriate behaviour. Evans hypothesised that men may therefore gravitate towards specialties that require less intimate touching of patients.

Summary

The principles and practices of nursing are ancient and in some part initiated and advanced by men. The number of men entering the nursing profession they helped create some 2,000 years ago remains stable. Compared to other professions, however, numbers still fall woefully short of desirable levels. Challenging societal prejudices and popular media images of the male nurse remains pivotal in recruiting and retaining male nurses.

References

Denny, E. and Earle, S. (2010) *Sociology for Nurses*, 2nd Edn. Cambridge: Polity Press.

Durgin, J.M. and Hanan, Z.I. (2009) *Pharmacy Practice for Technicians*, 4th Edn. New York: Delmar Cengage Learning.

Ellis, J.R. and Hartley, C.L. (2012) *Nursing in Today's World: Trends, Issues and Management*, 10th Edn. Baltimore, MD: Lippincott, Williams & Wilkins.

Evans, J.A. (2002) Cautious caregivers: Gender stereotypes and the sexualisation of men nurses' touch. *Journal of Advanced Nursing* 40(4): 441–448.

Finkelman, A. and Kenner, C. (2010) *Professional Nursing Concepts: Competencies for Quality Leadership*, 2nd Edn. Burlington, MA: Jones & Bartlett Learning.

McDonald, L. (2009) *Florence Nightingale: Extending Nursing*. Ontario, Canada: Wilfred Laurier University Press.

Middleton, J. (2014) Workforce issues hinder next generation of nurses, www.nursingtimes.net/opinion/editors-comment/workforce-issues-hinder-next-generation-of-nurses/5067873.article (accessed 17 July 2014).

Mohammed, J. (2010) On the lookout for men. *Nursing Standard* 26(30): 64.

Nursing and Midwifery Council (2008) *Statistical Analysis of the Register 1 April 2007 to 31 March 2008*. London: Nursing and Midwifery Council.

O'Lynn, C. (2013) *A Man's Guide to a Nursing Career*. New York: Springer.

Stokowski, L.A. (2012) Just call us nurses: Men in nursing. *Medscape*, 16 August, www.medscape.com/viewarticle/768914 (accessed 17 July 2014).

Traynor, M. (2013) *Nursing in Context: Policy, Politics, Profession*. Basingstoke: Palgrave Macmillan.

Useful web link

American Assembly of Men in Nursing: http://aamn.org.

Chapter 3

Misconceptions of nursing

Jon Harrison

Since becoming a nurse lecturer, I have always been intrigued and often amazed at how many student nurses, both on arrival and throughout their training, seem to not know what to expect when undertaking a nursing course at university. Why is this? Well, it is suggested that misconceptions of nursing held by the general public (and therefore you as a prospective nursing student) often conflict with the reality of nursing.

This chapter will explore these misconceptions further and then go on to discuss the reasons why prospective student nurses – like you perhaps – come to the course without really knowing what you are letting yourself in for. The final part of the chapter will then set out the main areas in which you can prepare further, thereby ensuring successful application to a course that should then harbour no surprises.

Why do you want to do nursing?

One of the most difficult questions that you may get asked is 'Why do you want to become a nurse?' Have you ever stopped to think about that question? Some find it hard to answer, because in truth, they just don't really know! Many nursing students I have asked tell me that they just know they 'have always wanted to be a nurse', often from a very young age, and they just want to care for and look after people. The desire to want to care for and help others therefore seems to be something that is innate – it has always been there and it is part of who you are.

The fact that you are reading this and feel that you are a caring individual who wants to help others, means that you are off to a good start. This is because these caring values that you possess are fundamental to the delivery of excellent nursing care. Because your values are intangible (meaning that you can't really touch or see them) they are very difficult things to influence or teach. We therefore need to make sure that you have these values before coming to do a nursing course. As a result, it is important that you demonstrate that you possess these values both within your application form, as well as during your interview.

Whilst possessing the right set of values and attitude is a crucial requirement in order to be accepted onto a nursing course, it is not the only thing you need to demonstrate if you want your application to be a successful one. Indeed, this is a scenario that I have often come across when I interview prospective student nurses. In most cases, it is evident that the applicant really wants to do nursing, and through their answers to my questions they can show that they have the caring and compassionate nature and values that are some of the vital ingredients of a good nurse. However, more often than not, the major stumbling block that the interviewee faces is the questions that relate to:

1 What is nursing?
2 What do nurses do?
3 What do you think you will be doing during the nursing course?

Before reading on, have a think about how you would answer these three questions if you were asked them in an interview.

Nursing is not like the media portrays it

So why is it that student nurses don't really know what to expect about the nursing course? Even for those that do feel they know what the course will entail, why do they then go on to find that the course wasn't what they had expected? The answers to these important questions often relate to the influences that may have had an impact on an individual's decision to do nursing. Have a think about what made you want to do nursing. We have already recognised that it is likely you will have a strong underpinning desire to want to help and care for others, but are there any other things that you can think of that have really made you want to do nursing? Perhaps you have had an experience in your life that has tipped the balance and confirmed to you that nursing is what you really want to do?

We know that many students who enter undergraduate nursing programmes develop their expectations and perceptions of nursing through a number of different influences. It

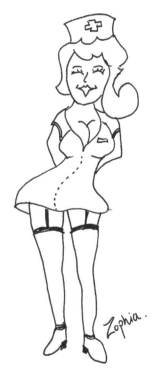

may be that prospective applicants have been involved in caring for a friend or family member, or they may have had their own experiences of being nursed themselves. It is also not uncommon for nursing applicants to already know other nurses, perhaps a friend or a member of their family.

One of the biggest influences, though, is the media. Have a think about the times you have seen nurses within the media and consider how these nurses have been portrayed. In the adverts and programmes that I have seen, it is not uncommon for nursing to be stereotypically portrayed as an all-female profession with the main duty being that of the doctor's hand-maiden. Nurses within hospital dramas are often portrayed as having less ability and are less academic than their medical colleagues. In addition, it is not uncommon within the media, for the image of nursing to be overly sexualised. Think how many times you have seen the stereotypical image of the 'naughty nurse' being used to sell products, such as shampoo for example.

Of course, not all programmes you see on the television are soap operas or dramas, and you will find some documentaries to be immensely informative and give a far more accurate reflection of what it is like to be a nurse. So whilst I am not suggesting you should ditch your *Casualty* or *Holby City* fix, just be aware that these types of programmes are unlikely to tell the whole story of what it is like to be a nurse. Let's look in more detail at a few more of the inaccuracies about nursing that can be found within the media.

For a start, nurses don't just work in hospitals. Other than the programme *Doctors*, all of the other healthcare-related serials that I can think of are all based in hospitals. Don't forget that nurses work in all sorts of different settings, many of which are outside of the hospital setting. If you have ever phoned NHS 111 (formerly NHS Direct) for example, it is likely that you would have spoken to a nurse. You will also find nurses in schools, GP surgeries, community health teams, and many midwives and health visitors will also have a nursing qualification. Further information relating to where you might work when you are a qualified nurse can be found in Part 5 of this book.

Related to the misconception of where they work, there is often a misunderstanding of who nurses work with. For example, the media seems to portray nurses' only role as caring for the sick, but actually the promotion of health and prevention of illness is just as important an aspect of nursing. Remember the old adage 'prevention is better than cure'.

When I have spoken with students about how nursing is portrayed within the media, they are often frustrated with the way in which nursing is promoted as a glamorous profession. We have all seen programmes where if the 'pretty' nurses are not chasing after doctors, they seem to do little more than sit around and look nice in their uniforms. The students that I have spoken to wanted me to make sure that you were aware that, despite all of the rewards it brings, nursing is not as glamorous as it is made out to be in the media. You will instead have to work very hard in a physically demanding role, dealing with difficult and sometimes unpleasant situations, including the handling of bodily fluids.

Nursing is not just physically demanding though – it can also be very emotionally challenging. Here again, hospital dramas tend to do little justice to the range of feelings that a nurse may have to deal with just in the space of one day. You can probably think of many times where you have seen people in hospital dramas recover miraculously after a few chest compressions, a couple of electric shocks and the application of some oxygen. Amazingly, you then see these characters happily sitting up in bed moments later. In reality though, sadly not everyone does get better, and this misconception – coupled with another unhelpful stereotype of nurses being 'angels' – means that the general public often find it difficult to understand that we cannot always save lives.

The reality is that you may nurse individuals who are reaching the end of their lives, perhaps prematurely, and this can be emotionally challenging. You will also care for others who are in great pain, both physically as well as mentally, and this too can be very testing. At the other end of the spectrum, however, most nurses will agree that there is no better feeling than seeing someone you have cared for get back to their 'normal' self. I still remember the look on children's faces as they bounced out of the ward with all their bags, balloons and cards, following the news that they could be discharged home. These children had been very unwell just a few days earlier and it is therefore particularly

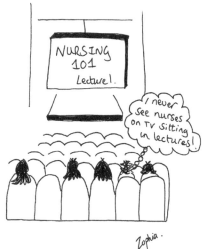

Zophia.

rewarding to know that you have helped someone feel a little better and that they could go on to achieve their full potential.

We have seen so far that there are many misconceptions of nursing, and it appears that when prospective nursing students consider what nursing is, more often than not, the influences around them tend to portray nurses in action – doing things that are practical and hands-on. Whilst on a day-to-day basis the media continues to show nurses at work in a hospital setting and personal experiences of hospitalisation or of caring for relatives may be at the forefront of people's minds, it seems rare that these influences portray student nurses having to think, problem solve, and study academic subjects within the university setting. It is therefore unsurprising that one of the common misconceptions of nursing, and indeed the nursing course, is that nursing is all about doing things that are hands-on and practical.

Nursing, and nurse education, is not just about 'doing things'

The common misconception that nursing is all about 'doing things' has led to a situation where many prospective nursing applicants are so consumed by the practical aspects of nursing that they underestimate the academic requirements related to the nursing course. Indeed, I have encountered a number of pre-registration nursing students who have been so surprised by the academic components of the course that they decided to leave the course.

This underestimation of the amount of academic work that you will be doing is perhaps not helped by another common misconception – this time relating to student life. Student nurses do not tend to fulfil the stereotypical view of what it is to be a student at university. The life of a student nurse is not one in which you attend a couple of lectures a week and then spend the remainder enjoying an exciting social life, or perhaps asleep. (To be honest though, no student life is like this really – not all the time anyway!)

Whilst there are some similarities with some of the other more traditional academic subjects, such as English, Maths or Philosophy for example, there are certainly some stark differences in terms of the student experience that you should be aware of. The most obvious difference relates to the fact that you will have to simultaneously fulfil the academic requirements whilst overcoming the complex demands of learning and working in the clinical practice environment.

I remember living in halls in my first year of the course, and my friends used to come round in the evening to see if I wanted to go and enjoy the best of the nightlife that Birmingham had to offer. Sometimes this was possible, and it was nice to feel like I had a 'student life' like the rest of my friends had, but sometimes I just had to say no – and that was hard! But the course I had chosen to do came with professional responsibilities that other courses simply do not have. So if I wasn't trying to finish an assignment, or revise for an exam, I probably had to get up at 5.30 a.m. so that I could get to an 'Early' shift on a Saturday morning.

It is important to remember that nursing will involve working both during the day and at night, during the week, at weekends – and when others are enjoying their holidays too! I still remember the first Christmas Day that I was due to work an early shift and arriving at the ward when all the children were opening their stockings. Whilst the rest of my family were enjoying the annual Christmas reunion, I was looking after sick children and their families, a hundred miles away from my Christmas lunch.

Shift work is not all bad though. As I worked 'long days' which means working four longer days rather than five, it meant that I would have three days off a week. It was really nice to be able to have that extra day off, to do what I wanted with. It is also one of the best feelings to finish your last night shift and travel home past everyone else on their way to work! (In case you were wondering, when you are qualified you do get paid extra for any work you do in what is termed as 'unsocial hours' – night shifts, weekend work and bank holidays.)

Addressing the misconceptions

It is important to address these misconceptions early on in your preparation to become a nurse, as expectations, both accurate and otherwise, have been shown to have close links with motivation, commitment and overall achievement. For example, if your expectations and values of the nursing course are subsequently upheld, then this is likely to fuel motivation, achievement and your commitment. Conversely though, if you find that aspects of the course are not like you thought they would be, then the result can be loss of motivation and underachievement, and this is where you may be putting yourself at risk of leaving the course.

Of course, it is not suggested that you will be able to prepare for everything, as no one can predict the future. Hopefully though, as you have been reading this, you have begun to identify some of your own thoughts and feelings about nursing and the nursing course. You should be in a position now, therefore, where you can start to address some of the misconceptions, and this book will take you through, one by one, the practical steps that you can undertake in order to be fully prepared for the application process, as well as starting the course itself.

The first step, it is suggested, is to really get your head around what you think nursing actually is. Chapter 1 has already explored a number of definitions of nursing, so reading this was definitely a good starting point. If you are interested, the RCN (2003) has produced a good document entitled 'defining nursing' which seeks to both define nursing, as well as help describe nursing to others. Part 2, Researching the fields of nursing, will give you a valuable insight into the various fields of nursing.

The next step is to ensure you are as fully prepared as possible for what clinical practice is like. I always find it concerning that many nurse applicants apply for the course without actually having any nursing experience at all. Remember, by choosing to undertake a nursing course, you are not only making the decision to go to university, you are also choosing a profession and a career that may be one that you work in for the rest of your working life. Would you buy a house without having a look round it first, or a car without taking it for a test drive? Clearly, having a lack of clinical experience puts you at risk of sharing some of the commonly held perceptions, or perhaps misconceptions, of what nursing entails. This is because without seeing it for yourself, you will find it very difficult to describe what nursing is actually like.

The final area that you should prepare yourself for relates to the theoretical and academic component of the course, as well as the university experience itself. As we have seen, student nurses are often surprised by both the amount of academic work they have to do, as well as what they actually have to study. I too remember being quite amazed (as well as a little threatened) by the number of 'ologies' that I attended lectures for in my first year – with physiology, pharmacology, pathology, sociology and psychology being just a few! It is therefore important that you read up about the subject areas that you will cover during the course, so at least you know what the different areas involve.

In addition to this, students often find that studying at university is quite different from learning in a school or college setting. In order to be successful in the academic parts of the course, it is also worth considering the study skills that you may need to develop further. Have a think about the ways in which learning and teaching approaches in university may be different from the experiences you have had so far, and then consider how you might go about addressing these differences. When I was a student, I remember really struggling with the first assignment that I had to write because I never really had to write one before. All I knew about assignment writing at this stage in the course was that the piece of work should have a beginning, a middle and an end! I had to therefore really develop my assignment-writing skills during my first term at university – and I learnt about critical analysis, developing an argument, use of evidence and the mysterious art of referencing.

Part 4, What and where you will learn, discusses the different aspects of studying within the university setting and explores some of the study skills that you will need to develop, such as academic writing, private reading, time management, asking questions in large groups and IT competence.

Remember, managing life whilst at university consists of more than just managing the course. This may be the first time, for example, that you are moving away from home, your parents and your friends. You may have to learn how to plan your finances, find somewhere to live, manage your new-found social life, make a meal for yourself and do your washing! Whilst it is not my intention to sound like your parents, it is important that you do prepare for these aspects of life outside the course, as problems in life can subsequently affect your performance within the course. Part 4 will explore further the ways in which you can prepare for and perhaps manage life in university and clinical placement, and deal with some of the stresses that you may find whilst being a student at university.

Summary

In this chapter, we have explored the reasons why you have chosen to do nursing. We have also considered the different influences that may have had an impact on your decision and discussed some of the misconceptions that can arise as a result of these. You should now be more aware about the requirements of the course and satisfied that nursing involves the mastery of theory and practice, both of which are of equal importance.

However, please don't forget that the experience you are about to have involves far more than just 'doing a nursing course'. By choosing to go to university to do nursing, you are choosing one of the most exciting rollercoaster rides of a course. There will be ups and downs, good times and bad, but ultimately if you have prepared well, you will find it to be one of the best experiences of your life. Not only will you emerge from the course with a professional as well as an academic achievement, you will have taken some giant steps in what will be a very rewarding career. I wish you all the best with that.

Reference

Royal College of Nursing (2003) *Defining Nursing*. London: RCN Publishing.

Further reading

Boyd, V. and McKendry, S. (2012) *Getting Ready for Your Nursing Degree: The StudySMART Guide to Learning at University*. Harlow: Pearson.

Elcock, K. (2012) *Getting into Nursing*. London: Sage.

Siviter, B. (2013) *The Student Nurse Handbook: A Survival Guide*, 3rd Edn. Edinburgh: Bailliere Tindall.

Useful web link

Royal College of Nursing: www.rcn.org.uk.

Part 2

Researching the fields of nursing

Chapter 4

The uniqueness of adult nursing

Judy Lewis-Basson and Cathy Poole

'Adult nursing' is a varied and exciting field because it deals with patients from the age of 16 years to the end of life. This is a wide age range which involves many different aspects of care. It also includes a wide spectrum of life events that people may experience – childbirth, marriage, job changes, redundancies, divorce, death of family members. All these are major events which may impact on a person's health, possibly exacerbating pre-existing conditions, or causing someone to present with new symptoms. Adult nurses deal with individuals with medical and surgical issues, patients with long-term conditions, the acutely ill, and emergency and accidental injuries, and they can undertake advisory and health-promotion roles.

The age range is of particular interest as there is currently an increasingly ageing population in the UK. The Office for National Statistics (ONS) state that the oldest age groups are the fastest growing and the number of people over the age of 85 is expected to more than double from 1.4 million in 2010 to 3.5 million in 2035. The number of people who have celebrated their 100th birthday is set to rise more than eightfold, from 13,000 in 2010 to 110,000 in 2035 (ONS 2011). This has, and will continue to have, an impact on the type of conditions that people are presenting with, and puts greater emphasis on the health-promotion role that an adult nurse will engage in. Health promotion is aimed at improving the quality of the patient's life and may be about taking medication regularly, or at the appropriate time, e.g. after meals. The patient may use an inhaler and, as they have aged, the technique they use may not be as effective. The nurse will need to review their technique and then advise on the correct method and the devices that can assist a patient to get an adequate 'puff'.

Key themes studied

Adult nursing, like the other fields, takes a holistic view of the patients. This means that the physical, psychological, sexual, social and spiritual aspects of the individual's well-being will be assessed, and the needs met (Leathard and Cook 2009). However, with the adult field, the first emphasis is with the physical. This does not mean that the other aspects are disregarded, but addressed after the physical needs have been met. For example an adult nurse is concerned about the physical appearance of their patient. This is assessed by using the ABCDE method. The nurse will systematically work through: Airway, Breathing, Circulation, Decreased consciousness, Everything else (Hill 2010). The assessments of these five areas will clarify the relative risk that the patient is classified at. When care has been given as appropriate, then the nurse will be concerned with the other elements of holism. The ABCDE assessment may assist with this. When observing the patient's airway and breathing the nurse will also observe how they looked. Did they look 'unkempt'? Were there signs that the patient may be dehydrated, e.g. dry lips? Were dentures well fitted? These are all key questions which, if left unanswered, may lead to the patient being malnourished whilst in hospital – for example, unable to eat because their mouth is sore due to ill-fitting dentures. The other aspects of holism are assessed, and referrals will be made to the relevant healthcare professional if an issue or problem is identified.

Adult nursing covers a wide age range when many changes may be occurring in people's lives. A patient may have dependants – husband, wife, children and their own parents – who may become more dependent on them. This may mean that stress levels could be very high in a patient who has a young family to look after and/ or elderly parents that they usually care for. Imagine you are in a hospital bed recovering from surgery or an illness and you are constantly worrying whether your children are being cared for properly etc. This would have a negative effect on your rehabilitation, as stress will affect the functioning of the bodily processes. A stressed patient will have problems sleeping, their diges-tion will slow down, wound healing will be delayed, appetite will be affected, etc. (Kosier *et al.* 2008). Ensuring that the social factors of a patient's history are taken into account is therefore of para-mount importance.

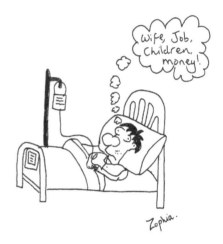

Practising nurse testimonials

Sam, a Clinical Nurse Specialist (CNS) for Pain Management, recounts an incident where social factors hampered a patient's recovery:

> A patient who had undergone a right knee replacement surgery ten days previously was referred to the Pain Management team. The lady was complaining of severe swelling and pain in her knee. The pain was preventing her from bending her knee and mobilising, consequently her discharge was delayed. I undertook a pain assessment on the lady and in a further discussion discovered that she has three cats at home. She was very anxious about the state of the cats. Her neighbour was going in once a day and she said that the cats were used to her being there all the time and talking to them. It transpired that since her surgery she had been refusing medication because she thought it might be addictive, constipate her and slow down her recovery, meaning she would have to stay in hospital longer. I reassured her and encouraged her to take regular pain relief (analgesia) whilst she was attempting to mobilise. I visited the lady two days later and she was mobilising well and preparing to be discharged. She was looking forward to seeing her cats!

Adult nursing is concerned with having the patient at the centre of their care. This means working with the inter-professional team, including: physiotherapists, doctors, dieticians (see Chapter 8, What skills and qualities are important?) and the patient's relatives/carers, with the patient at the centre. Patient-centred care facilitates a partnership, encourages involvement in decision making, and reaches a shared understanding of the patient's health status. The adult nurse is the linchpin in this process, being the member of the team who has the most contact with the patient and their relatives/carers. Therefore they need to be very understanding to the patient's feelings, ideas, needs and expectations (Abdelhadin and Drach-Zahavy 2012). This is demonstrated by being the patient's 'advocate' and supporting the patient to have the best possible health outcomes (NMC 2008).

Student Nurse Jane has provided a reflective account (see Gibbs 1998) of being a patient's advocate:

It was a first placement on an older adult ward and I was asked to attend a multi-disciplinary team meeting regarding one of the patients that I had been caring for with my mentor. The meeting took place in the ward office and the physiotherapist, occupational therapist, dietician, doctor, social worker, my mentor and I were present. The discussion began and the main issue was the lady's discharge to a nursing home to become a permanent resident. I had talked with the patient whilst giving care to her on many occasions and she had been very adamant that she did not want to give up her home. She had lived there for many years, raising her family. It was obviously full of memories. I informed the meeting what the lady had shared with me. After some debate the discharge plans were changed to put support in for her care in her own home.

I was very nervous at first voicing my concerns on behalf of the patient, but as I started to talk the staff listened to me and that encouraged me to carry on. I thought they might think, 'Who does she think she is?' as I was only a first year, but they didn't appear to.

I was very excited about the outcome and hoped that the patient would be as well. I thought that I had done my best for the patient as I had worked on her behalf as her advocate.

What I consider 'bad' about the situation was that the team members seemed to assume that because the patient was fairly elderly she would want to give up her home and be cared for in a nursing home. No one seemed to have discussed this with her prior to the meeting. What was good about the situation was that I knew the patient's wishes because I had discussed this with her and the team were willing to listen to me on the patient's behalf.

Analysing this event I think that more input from the patient should have been sought by members of the team prior to the meeting. Also I consider that it should have been acceptable for the patient to attend the meeting. No one seemed to ask her if she wanted to. Maybe documentation to be used prior to a multi-disciplinary team meeting could be put in place as a checklist, so that this situation does not occur again.

In conclusion I was pleased with my actions within this event and am glad I found the courage to speak up, although I was very scared – I would have more courage next time. I realise how important it is for nurses to be the patient's advocate, especially as we spend the most time with patients out of the members of the inter-professional team.

Within the adult field the nurse is required to perform a wide range of practical skills and may undertake many procedures on a daily basis. This will vary depending on the patient's diagnosis and condition. These skills include 'essential skills' such as taking the patient's observations, temperature, pulse, respirations and blood pressure, to the more complex skills, such as wound dressings, undertaking electrocardiography (ECG), female urinary catheterisation and passing a nasogastric (feeding) tube. As adult nursing is fairly 'hands on', including many clinical skills that the patients may require, it is a challenge to undertake these and maintain an individual's dignity, privacy and self-esteem. Depending on where an adult nurse is practising they may frequently catheterise a patient or pass a nasogastric tube. Both these procedures may drastically affect the patient's perception of their body image and cause them stress and anxiety. It is paramount that the adult nurse addresses these issues.

The skills that an adult nurse should possess are not just to do with dexterity but also personal traits. Good communication skills are obviously essential (Part 3 has more information on the personal traits you will need as a nurse). An adult nurse is in a very privileged position and will be involved in situations where patients share their innermost thoughts, feelings and fears which they may not have divulged to another person. This demands sensitivity and tact from the nurse to respond professionally and be able to meet the needs of that person. A sense of humour is also an asset – and can help to brighten the patients' lives as well!

The adult nurse will gain a huge insight into the lives of people, especially those of the ageing population, along with their values and beliefs. This can be a very rich experience – but the nurse always needs to be respectful, remembering what the older adult may have achieved in their life. A third-year nursing student, Emily, aged 24, was horrified at first to be placed in a nursing home for a clinical placement, considering that the care would be very 'basic' and not what she should be doing in her qualifying year. However afterwards she reflected on her experience:

> It was one of the best experiences I have had over the three years. The residents were mostly over 75 years. They were surrounded by their memorabilia, pictures of them in their youth, their families, certificates they may have won, medals, etc. It really made me appreciate who they had been and what they were, rather than when I see them in a hospital gown in a hospital bed! This experience has made me respect the older adults far more and nurse them with a greater consideration.

Being non-judgemental is a fundamental part of all nursing practice; but it may be quite a challenge for nurses in the adult field, for many reasons. To see a person suffer health consequences because of their poor choices of lifestyle (poor nutritional intake, smoking, alcohol intake) when they are cognitively able to make rational decisions can be frustrating for the practitioner. The individual may be seriously damaging their health and drastically shortening their lifespan, but may ignore health advice. This often leads to recurrent hospitalisation, which may affect not only the individual, but their families as well. Attempting to educate the patient regarding lifestyle choices and how to overcome barriers should be the nurse's main aim, but respecting the patient's choice with their ultimate decision, however hard for the nurse, must be done.

Adult nurses can work in a variety of settings. Box 4.1 shows some examples. Other settings may be pharmaceutical companies (usually as researchers), industry (occupational health settings), cruise ships, long-term care facilities, military facilities, and even refugee camps. Some nurses may also advise and work as consultants in the healthcare, insurance,

---

Box 4.1 Examples of hospital and community placements

Hospital

Accident and Emergency
Cardiac rehabilitation
Outpatients
Private hospitals
Operating theatres
Orthopaedic wards
Oncology (cancer) units
Renal (kidney) units

Community

Hospices
GP surgeries
Prisons
Community nurse
Walk-in health centres
School nursing
Retirement homes

---

or legal industries. Nurses can work full-time or part-time, and many work on a per diem basis or as travelling nurses. There is therefore a variety of areas that adult nurses can find themselves in during the course of their careers. More information about jobs and nursing around the globe can be found in Part 5.

Practice nurses working in GP surgeries undertake roles such as treating minor injuries, taking blood samples, health screening, family planning and promoting healthy lifestyles.

Prioritising care and decision making are essential facets of nursing care, and the adult nurse needs to be able to do these skilfully to enable patients to realise their best health outcomes. The role of the adult nurse is to promote health and well-being in their patients and assist them to have the best quality of life for them. Patients may be living with a long-term condition such as diabetes Type 1 or asthma, therefore the nurse will be required to educate and empower patients to realise how to make the best lifestyle choices to improve their life. Individuals may require more support at different times in their lives. This may not be age-related – it could be situational – therefore the assistance a person requires needs to be assessed on a dependence/independence continuum. An adult nurse will assess a patient to see where they are on this continuum and how much assistance they may need. Depending on the patient's situation they may fluctuate along this continuum, requiring frequent evaluation of their need for assistance. The 'Activities of living' (McCrae 2012) is a tool frequently used to assess adults. The aspects covered (see Box 4.2) such as breathing, sleeping, eating, etc. are assessed, with the dependence continuum as a measure of how

---

Box 4.2 Activities of living

Communication
Elimination
Eating and drinking
Maintaining a safe environment
Sleeping
Breathing

Washing and dressing
Controlling body temperature
Death and dying
Mobilisation
Working and playing
Expressing sexuality

much input the individual may require from the healthcare team. If a person has suffered trauma from a road traffic accident they may be very dependent at their time of admission to hospital. However, after the appropriate treatment has been delivered they may swiftly move along the continuum back to their original state of independence. This may contrast to a person who is very dependent with all needs prior to admission (Kara 2007).

As an adult student nurse you will gain experience in a variety of clinical settings. James, an adult student nurse in his 2nd year, provides his thoughts following a clinical placement on a spinal unit:

> I was very nervous on my first day on the spinal unit. It was a 20-bedded unit and all the patients were on the specially adapted beds so that they could be turned frequently to alleviate the pressure and reduce the risk of tissue damage. The patients were dependent on the nurses for all their needs. However there were certain tasks that they could still perform themselves. I wanted to do as much as I could for them but soon realised that to maintain their dignity and promote their independence I needed to encourage them to do as much as they could for themselves. I found this hard, as I felt I should be doing everything, but understood that it is a big part of the patient's successful rehabilitation.

There are many career prospects for the registered adult nurse; one of these is the role of the Clinical Nurse Specialist (CNS). A CNS is a registered nurse who has gained specialist knowledge and skill through theory, practice and on-the-job instruction. There are many CNSs in practice currently and they work in all the areas where an adult nurse may practise. The 'CNS for Diabetes' role includes providing clinical leadership in diabetic education and nursing, as well as providing clinical advice to nurses, doctors and other professionals. In addition, the CNS will participate in the development and facilitation of new procedures, techniques and protocols for a diabetic service. Another long-term condition which has a distinct CNS role is epilepsy. For most adults, the outlook is very good. With the help of adult nurses and the inter-professional team, symptoms can usually be controlled using medicines known as anti-epileptic drugs (AEDs). It can take some time to find the right type and correct dose of AED before seizures can be controlled. CNSs help the sufferers to gain a clear understanding of epilepsy, and with good management of seizures, the risk of sudden unexplained death in epilepsy can be minimised.

Alternative entry routes into adult nursing

There is an option to become an adult nurse via the armed forces. This is known as 'defence nursing'. Defence nursing is really an overarching term which is used to define the nursing capabilities which are supported by the Royal Air Force, the Army and the Royal Navy. (All the information contained in this section has been sourced from the relevant Services' websites which are an invaluable source of information for those would-be defence nursing students.) Collectively, the three uniformed Services are known as the Defence Medical Services (DMS). The role of the DMS is to promote, safeguard and reinstate the health of service personnel, to guarantee that they are medically fit and prepared to go wherever they are required across the world, which is known as being 'fit for task' (MoD 2012).

In order to become a nurse within the armed forces you are required to pass the relevant entry criteria/checklist for the relevant armed force, as well as the university student nurse entry criteria. The university student nurse entry criteria are explained in detail in Chapter 9.

Via the Royal Air Force

This route allows you to join the Royal Air Force (RAF) and first complete a 10-week basic training programme. You then continue to be employed and paid by the RAF as a student nurse, during which time you undertake the fully funded 3-year full-time BSc (Hons) in Nursing. This nurse training is completed at Birmingham City University (www.bcu.ac.uk/) alongside civilian adult student nurses. You will undertake clinical placements in both civilian and service areas. Before you consider this route into adult nursing, however, it is worth looking at the 'eligibility check' on the RAF website (www.raf.mod.uk/recruitment/how-to-apply/eligibility-check/).

This site includes details about the following:

- Nationality and residency
- Age requirements
- Educational requirements
- Fitness requirements
- Health requirements
- Background checks
- Disqualifying factors.

One of the unique features of training as an adult student nurse in the RAF is the fact that you will be paid during your training. This pay is currently (October 2014) £17,945 during your first year at university, and will rise to £21,259 in your final year. You will also be entitled to other benefits, as identified in Box 4.3.

You must remember that joining the RAF is a big commitment. You are required to join for a minimum of 9 years initially, or for 22 years ('open engagement'). You can however leave at any time after your 9 years, by handing in your resignation. During your nurse training you will also be required to take part in service-related activities such as fitness, parades and meetings. On completion of your three years' undergraduate nurse training you will graduate and commence your nursing career as an RAF Registered Nurse (Adult), as an Acting Corporal. As a nurse in the RAF you will be part of the Princess Mary's Royal Air Force Nursing Service (PMRAFNS). Further information about becoming an adult nurse

---

Box 4.3 RAF benefits

Educational support	Healthcare
Sponsorship and scholarships	Time abroad
Room and board	Discounts
Holidays	Bonuses
Sports	Pension
Gym	Maternity and paternity benefits

via the RAF can be found at www.raf.mod.uk/recruitment/roles/medical-and-medical-support/student-nurse-adult.

Via the Army

This route allows you to join the Army and complete a 14-week Phase 1 military training at Pirbright or Winchester, where you will gain basic soldiering skills and fitness. Then you will be able to start your adult student nurse training. As with the other Services, your

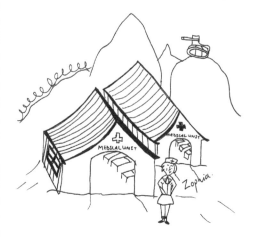

undergraduate nurse training will be undertaken at Birmingham City University with civilian student nurses, and you will gain a BSc in Nursing. The three-year course is a mix of theory and practice as defined by the Nursing and Midwifery Council (2010). Luckily, as with the other Services, you will be paid while you study. More details on Army pay can be found at www.army.mod.uk/join/25652.aspx.

When you qualify as a Registered Nurse you will have the opportunity to travel and work overseas in MoD Hospital Units, Medical Centres or Medical Regiments. Wherever the Army is across the globe, registered nurses are always required to meet the nursing needs of injured persons, maintain their health and prevent illness. As a nurse in the Army you will be part of the Queen Alexandra's Royal Army Nursing Corp (QARANC). Further information about becoming an adult nurse via the Army can be found at www.army.mod.uk/rolefinder/role/228/student-nurse.

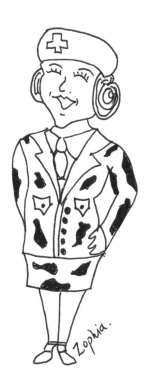

Via the Royal Navy

This route allows you to join the Royal Navy as part of the Queen Alexandra's Royal Naval Nursing Service (QARNNS) as an adult student nurse. As with the other armed forces, as an adult student nurse you will spend your first three years with other civilian and Service adult student nurses at Birmingham City University. You will be based at the university's Defence School of Health Care Studies during which time you will undertake a BSc in Nursing. In readiness for becoming a Naval Nurse you will be required to gain clinical experience in civilian hospitals and in a field hospital, or at sea on the RFA *Argus*, the Royal Navy's 'Primary Casualty Receiving Facility'.

Before you consider this route into adult nursing, however, it is worth looking at the Royal Navy website to review their eligibility criteria (www.royalnavy.mod.uk/careers/how-to-join/apply/~/media/3cd18a33f8 0c4133967cfc4351756df6.ashx). This site includes details about the following:

- Age
- Restrictions by gender
- Height and weight
- Tattoos
- Body piercing
- Nationality
- Residency
- Medical standards
- Eyesight
- Temporary conditions
- Contact with the Police or a prosecuting agency
- Drug and substance misuse
- Financial commitments – debt and bankruptcy
- Academic requirements
- Fitness standards.

As with the other Services, entering nursing as a student nurse will also require you to meet the same UCAS entry criteria.

When qualified as a Naval Nurse you will have the opportunity to work at sea and on shore, helping to provide nursing support to Royal Navy and Royal Marines personnel across the globe. Further information about becoming an adult nurse via the Royal Navy can be found at www.royalnavy.mod.uk/careers/role-finder/roles/nursestudent#.

As a qualified adult registered nurse it is probable that you will be posted to a secondary care unit. These secondary care units in the UK are provided in conjunction with the National Health Service at the Royal Centre for Defence Medicine (in Birmingham) and Ministry of Defence Hospital Units (in Frimley Park, Portsmouth, Derriford and Northallerton).

Summary

Adult nursing offers many opportunities and the chance to meet a diverse patient group. There are challenging situations and ones in which patients, carers and the nurse need to have courage and commitment, but this field offers rich rewards to the dedicated practitioner. It is wonderful to witness the patient being discharged after recovering from major surgery or a trauma. Also, to see someone with a long-term condition (rheumatoid arthritis, asthma, chronic obstructive airway disease, diabetes) managing to get a good quality of life and be independent is fantastically rewarding. There are also many career options for the registered adult nurse and different areas where they are being asked to practise.

Remember you can also become an adult student nurse via the three armed forces and gain your BSc in Nursing but be mindful that as a registered nurse you may be deployed to conflict areas and find yourself assisting with humanitarian efforts. Whichever route you take to enter adult nursing you will quickly realise that the career opportunities are widespread and varied.

References

Abdelhadi, N. and Drach-Zahavy, A. (2012) Promoting patient care: work engagement as a mediator between ward service climate and patient-centred care. *Journal of Advanced Nursing* 68(6): 1276–1287.

Gibbs, G. (1988) *Learning by Doing: A Guide to Teaching and Learning Methods*. London: Further Education Unit.

Hill, K. (2010) Rapid assessment of the acutely ill patient. *Nursing in Critical Care* 15(4): 223.

Kara, M.J. (2007) Using the Roper, Logan and Tierney Model in care of people with COPD. *Clinical Nursing* 16(7B): 223–233.

Kosier, B., Erb, G., Berman, A., Snyder, S., Lake, R. and Harvey, S. (2008) *Fundamentals of Nursing: Concepts, Process and Practice*. London: Pearson Education.

Leathard, H.L. and Cook, M.J. (2009) Learning for holistic care: Addressing practical wisdom (phronesis) and the spiritual sphere. *Journal of Advanced Nursing* 65(6): 1318–1327.

McCrae, N. (2012) Whither nursing models? The value of nursing in the context of evidence-based practice and multidisciplinary health care. *Advanced Nursing* 68(1): 222–229.

Ministry of Defence (2012) *Defence Medical Services*. www.gov.uk/defence-medical-services (accessed 10 October 2014).

Nursing and Midwifery Council (2008) *The Code: Standards of Conduct, Performance and Ethics for Nurses and Midwives*. London: Nursing and Midwifery Council.

Nursing and Midwifery Council (2010) *Standards for Pre-Registration Nursing Education*. London: Nursing and Midwifery Council.

Office for National Statistics (2012) www.ons.gov.uk/ons/index (accessed 9 March 2014).

Further reading

Castledine, G. and Close, A (2009) *Oxford Handbook of Adult Nursing*. Oxford: Oxford University Press.

Moore, C. (2006) The transition from student to qualified nurse: A military perspective. *British Journal of Nursing* 15(10): 540–542.

Richards, A. and Edwards, S.L (2012) *A Nurse's Survival Guide to the Ward*, 3rd Edn. Edinburgh: Churchill Livingstone.

Royal College of Nursing (2013) Defence Nursing Forum Membership Leaflet. Publication Code: 004 487, www.rcn.org.uk (accessed 10 October 2014).

Siviter, B. (2013) *The Student Nurse Handbook: A Survival Guide*, 3rd Edn. Edinburgh: Bailliere Tindall.

Useful web links

Army: www.army.mod.uk/join/join.aspx

Birmingham City University: http://moodle.bcu.ac.uk/health/course/view.php?id=3489

Defence Medical Services: www.gov.uk/defence-medical-services

NHS Careers: www.nhscareers.nhs.uk/explore-by-career/nursing/careers-in-nursing/adult-nursing

Nursing and Midwifery Council: www.nmc-uk.org/Documents/Standards/The-code-A4-20100406.pdf

Royal Air Force: www.raf.mod.uk/careers

Royal College of Nursing: www.rcn.org.uk/development/students/careers/advice

Royal College of Nursing Defence Nursing Forum: www.rcn.org.uk/development/nursing_communities/rcn_forums/defence

Royal Navy: www.how2become.com/royal-navy.

Chapter 5

The uniqueness of children's and young people's nursing

Lisa Abbott, with Cathy Poole

When I was a student children's nurse, back in 1994, I entered the ward for my first ever shift. It was 7 a.m., the middle of winter and pitch black outside. As I walked through the ward down towards the nursing station, I heard the sound of the opening song to *The Lion King* movie. Wow, I thought, this is where I want to be, I had expected a much more sterile environment, but there were pictures and toys everywhere, children playing and talking with their parents, who had camp beds beside them. The children seemed to be having fun, despite their illnesses, injuries or pain. The ward seemed to be organised, everyone looked busy and had a job to do, but still found the time to be welcoming and friendly! Children's nursing was the best decision I have ever made and one which has given me a very rewarding, sometimes challenging, but immensely satisfying career.

Children's nursing is a broad term that covers many age groups from 0–18. For the purpose of this book, we will refer to all these age groups as children, yet it must be remembered that this could mean small babies or young people entering adulthood. Children are not just small adults – they are a diverse group, varying in so many different ways:

- Age
- Stage of development
- Weight
- Physiology
- Size and shape
- Intellectual ability
- Emotional response
- Psychological maturity.

(Advanced Life Support Group 2011: 7)

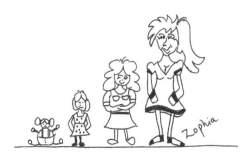

To be able to care for this unique group you need to be able to adapt yourself, to interact at the right level for the child, and acknowledge their varied needs. The types of illnesses and injuries that children encounter are potentially different to adults, and the way they respond physiologically and emotionally is also different. Children can get sick quickly but they can recover speedily, without the psychological attachment of illness. For example a child with a fever will look poorly and not interact much, and as soon as the temperature is reduced the child will appear to instantly feel better and want to play. A child is the centre of the family's life and the family is the centre of the child's life – it is therefore an absolute priority that the family are involved in all aspects of the child's care.

What is children's and young people's nursing?

Here is a quick guide to the history and development of children's nursing. Just 170 years ago there were no children's hospitals in Britain. During this time, in London alone, there were 21,000 deaths per year of children under 10 (Glasper and Charles-Edwards 2002). The philosophy then was 'Who could care better for a child than their mother?' which in some ways is sensible – and does recognise the importance of the family in a child's care. However, in 1852, the first Children's Hospital was opened in Great Ormond Street, London. One of the founding aims of this hospital was that children needed to be nursed by those who are educated in the management of children and infants during illness. In 1859 Florence Nightingale stated that 'It is a real test of a nurse whether she can nurse a sick infant' – clearly recognising the complexities of nursing children. In the nineteenth century, the philosophy surrounding children's nursing was based around the needs of the child, including warmth, understanding, love and the importance of keeping the child happy (Glasper and Charles-Edwards 2002; Davies and Davies 2011: 13).

This philosophy was set to change, and in the early twentieth century a more objective approach to caring for children developed, which was less care-driven and more disease-oriented. It prioritised the role of the nurse and doctors over the needs of the family. In fact, parents were almost excluded completely from care, only being allowed to visit for perhaps thirty minutes per week, and then not allowed to hold their child! The traumatic effects of this separation of families and their children are well documented through research conducted by Robertson and Bowlby in the 1950s (Bretherton 1992).

In 1959, the Ministry of Health published the Platt Report. This signalled the importance of children's nurses having specialist education and training. It made many recommendations which have led to the way we deliver care today. These recommendations brought back the importance of the family in the care of the child. The Report recommended that separation should be avoided, and that children should be cared for in cheery environments with facilities for play. Davies and Davies (2011: 22) suggest this move to family-centred care brought love back to children's nursing. And I say thank goodness – I don't think I could bear to nurse children in an environment without their parents and without play!

A child's right to good healthcare, survival, growth and protection, and to have a happy childhood may seem obvious, but in fact it is only in the last 25 years that these rights have become more established. In 1989, the United Nations Convention on the Rights of the Child clearly spelt out that children should have the right to protection, to good healthcare provision and to be able to participate in decision making about their lives (www.unicef.org.uk/UNICEFs-Work/Our-mission/UN-Convention).

Furthermore the Children Act 1989 and 2004 gave children protection under British law, and defined that 'The child's welfare must be paramount'. In 2004 the Department of Health published the National Service Framework for Children, Young People and Maternity Services. This provides a set of standards, detailing the care that should be delivered, based upon recommendations from various public inquiries, which included the following:

- The Victoria Climbié Inquiry report by Lord Laming (2003)
- The Bristol Royal Infirmary Inquiry (2001)
- The National Service Framework (2004)

In 1919 the Nurses Registration Act provided a professional register for general (adult) nurses governed by the General Nurses Council. There was controversy about the necessity of a register for children's nurses, as it was the belief by some that anyone could care for children. However, eventually it was agreed to open a supplementary register for children's nurses. Although its value did diminish for a while, it is now back in full strength. In 1989, direct entry into the field of Children's Nursing was formalised through professional registration via the United Kingdom Central Council, now known as the Nursing and Midwifery Council (NMC) (Glasper and Charles-Edwards 2002; Davies and Davies 2011: 21–22).

Children's nursing is an exciting, demanding and fulfilling career, with a wide range of opportunities available to you. To nurse children, you need to have some special qualities. First and foremost you need to like, if not love children, and want to make a positive difference to their lives, through delivery of nursing care, advice or health promotion (Rushforth 2008). You need to be able to connect with children of all ages and stages of development. You need to have a good sense of humour, and the ability to have fun whilst retaining your professionalism.

Children have unique needs which develop and change as they grow older and go through various stages of development and maturity (sometimes called 'transitions'). The range of ages you may look after is wide, from a tiny premature baby to an 18-year-old adolescent, so you can imagine how their needs will change as they reach various developmental milestones.

You need to be skilful in talking, listening and recognising non-verbal signals sensitively with these varying ages. Sometimes you have to use the detective work of observation and deduction to discover what is wrong with your patient. This is because children either cannot or do not always describe their symptoms well – either because they do not have the language to do so, or because fear and pain may be stopping them. For example, a toddler who cannot talk cannot tell you where the pain is, and an older child may not want to tell you where the pain is, for fear it may become worse or fear that he might get an injection!

When communicating with children it is always important to be honest, to gain their trust and respect. Children seem to be able to detect a lie, even a little one, and this could mean you lose that child's trust. Then they may not open up and share how they are feeling with you or they may become less willing to comply with the treatment they are receiving (Siviter 2013).

Nursing children could incorporate a wide variety of conditions – of a medical nature (such as a chest infection) or of a surgical nature (a tonsillectomy, for example). Illnesses can be 'acute', which means they happen for a short period of time, such as appendicitis, or they can be 'chronic' which means they have long-lasting effects, such as cystic fibrosis. You may also care for children with learning disabilities such as Down Syndrome or with mental health problems – depression, for example.

Children can become very poorly and require intensive care, either post-surgery (due to worsening illness such as bronchiolitis) or suddenly, following an incident (such as a road traffic collision). Dealing with parents whose child is critically ill can be an emotionally charged job. It involves ensuring that the right amount of information is delivered to keep them well informed and providing the right amount of emotional support, as well as providing the best quality care. Having a sick child is probably the most stressful thing for a parent and family to cope with. People's coping strategies are different – some may be angry and give quite direct comments to you, whilst others may be crying in the corner. It is your job to intuitively know the right amount of support to offer and not to take offence with the angry parent, but understand their concerns. Helping families cope with this experience is a crucial part of your role, placing families at the centre of the care and enabling them to express themselves as best they can (NHS 2012).

You cannot cure everybody, and at times children may die, either unexpectedly, or they may have a terminal illness which leads to their death. This is of course an untimely tragedy, and enough to make anybody cry. Therefore if a child in your care does die, it is OK to show your emotions and to cry with parents. It shows your humanity and your ability to empathise with the parents and family. It would be easy to fall apart and become very emotional, yet it is important that we try to remain strong for the child and their family, providing appropriate support in every way possible, to ensure dignified end-of-life care.

Often people say 'I couldn't be a children's nurse as it would be too upsetting, especially when children die.' Of course the death of a child is regarded as one of the most traumatic events that families have to deal with. However, as children's nurses, as part of a caring compassionate team, you will endeavour to ensure that children and their families faced by death will be fully informed, supported and involved in decisions relating to end-of-life care (terminal care). This support may include pain and symptom management, access to children's hospices, access to specialist nursing services – for example, Macmillan Nurses – and help with directing bereaved families to specialist bereavement trusts and charities. Aiding a child and family faced with death in an empathetic, kind and gentle professional manner can be as rewarding as seeing a very sick child bounce back to health and be discharged home. But the day that you no longer feel upset and emotional at the loss of a child you have cared for should be the time you hang up your nurse's uniform and change careers.

When children are hospitalised due to illness or for investigation, it is normal practice for parents to stay with their child during this time. In fact, children's wards on the whole allow open visiting, including brothers and sisters, grandparents, school friends and anyone who is special to the child – even pets. This can lessen the anxiety surrounding admission to hospital and provide a sense of normality to the child which can decrease any sense of isolation.

Children's nurses understand the importance of the surrounding family, and successful collaboration, known as 'family-centred care', can have a huge impact on the ability of the child to

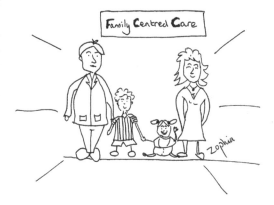

cope with their illness, because children are cared for best by their own parents (Nursing and Midwifery Council 2010a). It is hoped by negotiating care with the child and family that some elements of normal routine can be maintained for the child, thus reducing the effects of the potentially frightening admission to hospital. Family know their child best, their normal routine, and how they react to various situations. It is really important that we use this 'insider' information to understand the child's normal behaviour pattern, and then if the child deteriorates we are able to detect this change quickly and initiate appropriate action.

As a children's nurse you may be providing care in a variety of different environments, for example:

- a children's hospital
- a children's ward in a district general hospital
- at the child's home, as a community children's nurse
- day care
- a hospice
- as a school nurse
- as a health visitor.

Although there are of course times when hospital admission is necessary, the best place to care for children, if at all possible, is in their home. Community Children's Nursing teams are now more established and there are options such as Hospital at Home for children with a variety of needs – for example a child requiring long-term support of their breathing via a machine, or more simply the management of a child with a fever. Nursing a child at home can provide a better recovery because it can avoid the anxiety and stress related to hospital admission. There can be more stimulation, leading to a more 'normal' child development. Children would get to be part of normal family events, such as birthdays and Christmas. Furthermore, the likelihood of hospital-acquired infections can be reduced (Davies and Davies 2011: 246). It can actually save the NHS considerable money, but it must be well managed – the nurses, family and carers need appropriate education, and there is a lot to organise in terms of equipment and staffing.

No matter where you care for children or what age they are it is important to ensure that they have their privacy and dignity at all times. Even though they are young, they still have the need for privacy, for example when getting dressed or having their nappy changed. It is important to involve the child and family in decisions about the care being given. This could be as simple as asking if it's OK to feel someone's pulse or as serious as gaining consent for an operation. Ethical and legal issues can create some dilemmas in children's nursing, especially where a child is deemed able to be involved in the decision-making process, yet their views may conflict with the views of the medical staff and parents. It is important to recognise the child's right to make their own decisions, and to speak up for them and respect their rights as much as possible.

As a children's nurse you will learn many clinical skills around medicines management, assessment, observation and prioritisation. For example, a key skill of the children's nurse is to ensure adequate nutrition – whether it is supporting a mother to breastfeed, giving a baby a bottle feed, feeding via a tube into the stomach, managing feeds delivered intravenously, or promoting healthy eating habits. Administering medicines to children is another vital component of the role of the nurse (and, as you can imagine, just getting a child to agree to take some medicine can be a challenge in itself).

Medicines management in children is complex, and requires good numerical ability. All medicine doses prescribed for children and young people are calculated using the patient's weight (and sometimes their body surface area). Liquid medicines (oral suspensions which most children prefer) come in a variety of drug solutions – Paracetamol suspension, for example, is available as 120 mg in 5 mL, or 250 mg in 5 mL. Therefore if your patient was prescribed 45 mg of Paracetamol you would need to calculate how many mL you would need to administer. Clearly, administering medicines safely to children and young people is not as simple as just giving two Paracetamol tablets.

When giving any medicine to a child it is important that you have a full understanding of the medicine you are about to administer, why you are giving it, and what the potential side effects might be. You must also give clear explanations to the child and family, gain consent to give the medicine and then document and monitor the effects. In many cases you will be asking the child's family or carers to actually administer medications on your behalf, your responsibility being to ensure that the child cooperates with their family. Children can and do sometimes refuse the medicines you want to give them, whether they are aged 2 or 12. Think now . . . How would you encourage children of different ages to take their medicines?

Children and their families, especially those coping with long-term illnesses, often know their condition inside out, and will quite possibly know more about it than you do! They may question the care you deliver, including the medicines you give. It is important to recognise and respect their experience, and learn from them about how to best care for their child.

You might be surprised to know that as a children's nurse you will become a teacher! This may be to colleagues and student nurses around you but in particular to children and their families. Here are some examples of the things you are likely to teach children and their families during your career:

- about their particular condition;
- you might teach and support a parent to care for their child;
- perhaps how to pass a feeding tube (nasogastric tube);
- how to give medicines effectively;
- how to recognise complications of treatment;
- how to give injections;
- how to perform kidney dialysis.

These are just a few of the examples, and it is probable that what and who you teach will be determined by the direction in which your nursing career takes you – you could even become a nurse lecturer!

It is impossible to talk about children's nursing without talking about play. Children use play to socialise, rehearse situations and learn. As children go through the stages of development they will use different types of play to learn. Imaginative play is perhaps the most fun stage. Children have amazing imaginations, and can pretend they are anywhere doing anything at any time! As a nurse, you can really harness the use of play to help children cope with their illness or injury.

Play enables children to develop coping strategies for the experience of being in hospital, and provides preparation for interventions to follow. For example, you could rehearse putting a bandage on a teddy bear before putting it on a child. This would allow them an understanding and control of what is going to happen next and therefore decrease anxiety related to interventions. It is amazing how blowing bubbles or a 'spot the difference' book can provide distraction therapy to enable children to endure procedures, such as having blood samples taken. We quite often use 'magic' cream, to help the pain of having a needle inserted; this numbs the skin and lessens the pain of the procedure, and can provide a more positive experience of what can sometimes be painful.

The recognition of a child's bravery is very important. I know as a mother, if my son or daughter falls over and grazes their knee, they can be in floods of tears, but as soon as I have acknowledged what has happened, said what a brave boy or girl and kissed it better, the tears stop. Even better is a plaster. Children love plasters – to them it is recognition they have an injury. After the kiss on the knee, the next question is often, Can I have a plaster? They will then show it off to their friends and family!

Children respond well to reward charts, so if you are having difficulty getting a child to take their medicine or eat their dinner, providing a reward in the form of a sticker on a chart can be very motivational. It is important to have an idea of current children's television characters, popular electronic games, current music and social networking, as these are things the child may relate to and they might make it easier for you to talk with them. Equally, you will need to be up to date with what adolescents like in terms of activities, music, television programmes, fashion – and, of course, their body image and teenage language, such as 'text speak'.

When in hospital, children of school age will still receive schooling, either at the bedside, or they can go to the hospital school. This provides some normality for children and attempts to keep them up to date with their schooling, so they don't get left behind their classmates. Being in hospital as a child does not necessarily mean that you are confined there. If children are well enough they may be allowed day trips out. For example, I know of children who have been dependent on oxygen or a breathing machine and potentially confined to hospital, but the nursing staff have striven to give those children the little treats in life. Organising appropriate support to enable the child and family to go on day trips out – simply to go around the block, out to the garden, play centre, the Disney store or even the Sealife Centre – are welcomed activities to the child and their family.

Children's nursing is a popular field but it is not an easy option. However, the satisfaction associated with helping to make a child better is immense, especially when a parent thanks you for what you have done!

Key themes studied

During your children's nurse training you will cover many topic areas. The NMC (2010b) laid out standards for pre-registration nurse training, which are based on the four domains of nursing, as shown in Box 5.1. (How these standards are delivered and monitored is explained in more detail in Part 4.)

Putting theory into practice

Fifty per cent of your course will be learning whilst out on clinical practice placements (practice experience). This will include a wide variety of areas, which will enable you to see

Box 5.1 NMC nursing domains

Domain 1 Professional values

Advocacy
Working in partnership
Child and family centred care
Empower children to express their views
Maintain and recognise children's rights and best interests
Learn about governing laws.

Domain 2 Communication and interpersonal skills

Take account of each child's individuality, including:

- Stage of development
- Ability to understand
- Culture
- Learning or communication difficulties

Communicate effectively with parents, carers and families
Use play
Communicate at appropriate level
Involve children and young people in decision making.

Domain 3 Nursing practice and decision making

Care for children in all settings
Take responsibility for safeguarding them
Use evidence-based practice and child-centred frameworks to assess, plan, implement and evaluate nursing care
Care planning and delivery must be informed by knowledge of pharmacology, anatomy, numeracy, physiology, pathology, psychology and sociology from infancy to young adulthood.

Domain 4 Leadership, management and team working

Health and social policies relating to children
Empower and enable young people
Use effective decision making in complex situations
Provide a smooth transition to adult services.

(Adapted from NMC 2010b: 40–48)

Box 5.2 Examples of clinical practice placements

Possible community placements

Community children's nurse
Health visitor
School nurse
Nursery school
Special school
Day centre
Children's hospice

Possible hospital-based placements

Medical wards
Surgical ward
Children's wards at district general hospitals
Out-patients
Day patients
Baby wards
Adolescent wards
Child and adolescent mental health services (hospital and community)
High dependency/Paediatric intensive care unit
Emergency department (A&E)

---

all aspects of children's nursing and help you to learn about the well child and the child during illness or injury. Box 5.2 provides some examples of where you may be allocated to spend time.

Student nurse testimonials

These are some testimonials from student child field nurses, about why children's nursing is so special.

> I feel that if children with medical conditions and illnesses find courage and determination to deal with what life throws at them, then how could I not support and encourage that? Children don't choose to be in hospital, so to be able to help them is priceless (and more rewarding than any pay packet) as we are enabling children to be children and not just an illness or condition.
>
> Gemma Grosvenor, 3rd year student nurse

> Children's nursing has always been special to me. You not only meet some amazing children of all ages with all sorts of conditions and receiving all different treatments, you

also get to meet some amazing parents/carers and families! Also what is so interesting is that children can become so ill but get better so quickly! It's so rewarding to see a child leave the ward back to their normal self and seeing a happy family!

Lucy Evans, 2nd year student nurse

Children's nursing enables a special insight into family life. We are fortunate to be able to be a part of the family's journey. We are there at special occasions such as birthday, Christmas, first words, first steps or even breathing unassisted or eating orally for the first time. We also share the family's highs and lows with them, we cry when they cry, we feel their pain, we feel pride and fear, we share a family's happiness, we want the best for their child and do all within our powers to ensure their child gets the best and highest possible care possible. Our work does not end at the door – we remember our patients' little faces for years to come and wonder what has become of them.

Sarah Gardner, 3rd year student nurse

Children's nursing is a dynamic yet challenging role to fulfil. It is so much more than looking after children! This role ensures parents, siblings, aunts, uncles, friends and the child are all involved in the situation and the care delivered, and that their needs are met. It is a special kind of nursing because we can fulfil and go beyond their expectations; we hold their hand through the difficult times and are a powerful advocate in what can be a frightening setting. Children's nursing is special because you are kept on your toes, challenged and rewarded all in the same day.

Victoria Lynne, 2nd year student nurse

I feel being a children's nurse is a special privilege. Being able to help a child and family through a difficult time, either seeing them grow and recover, or sadly help in any way you can in sad circumstances. Having the honour that you may be remembered for the rest of their life or, in my case, the reason they grow up to want to help children themselves.

Holly Phipps, 3rd year student nurse

Children's nurses are in a league of their own. They possess a special ability to always put on a happy smile, even when there's not a lot to smile about. They adapt to each child's individual needs and adapt the care they give. They are the ones who gain the children's trust and make them feel secure in what for most is an alien environment. Most important of all they are devoted and care about each child they treat – they take care of our country's future.

Amie Heycock, 2nd year student nurse

Practising and newly qualified nurse testimonials

We try really hard every day to show compassion, respect, commitment, courage and trust to the children, families and colleagues to the best of our ability. No two days are ever the same. People ask 'How can you be a children's nurse? It would make us cry.' Those of us who have that honour do not feel like that. We are there to comfort those who are crying. Some days are great when we teach families to be independent and go home with help of community teams. Some children are unable to go home, or do not survive. This is not a failing. We try to give the best care with the help of the whole team and hospice staff.

> Elaine Sexton, Clinical Nurse Specialist, Nutritional Care

One thing that I always think of is that as a children's nurse we are entrusted with a parent's greatest gift – their child. What greater honour or privilege could there be?

No matter what adversity a child faces, they will always try to smile, and a smile from a child can brighten up the worst days, make you cry, make you laugh, make it all worthwhile.

> Ian Coxon, Senior Charge Nurse, Emergency Department

Children's nursing is special because it is the only job where you can do something very small that makes an impact on someone for life – where your reward costs nothing, but means the world!

You might be giving medication, smiling at a child in the lift, making a cup of tea, or supporting families through a crisis, but for that you get a giggle, a smile, tears of relief and acceptance or a thank you, and that tells me as a nurse that, whatever the outcome, I have made a difference.

Being a children's nurse means that you live in reality every day – children can't hide their feelings or emotions. Every day I am inspired and reminded that I am fortunate to be in the position I am.

> Lisa Gilks, Senior Sister, Emergency Department

I think it's a privilege that parents allow me to care for the most precious thing they have. It's special to think you can touch the lives of these amazingly brave kids and families' lives.

> Rachel Morrison, Paediatric Intensive Care Unit

Watching the relief slowly spread across a parent's face when you tell them their child's condition is improving fills me with joy every time.

> Phil Wilson, Lead Nurse, KIDS Intensive Care and Decision Support

Summary

As you can see, it takes a special person to be able to provide holistic family-centred care to children and their families, enabling them to be part of the care delivery and decision-making process, whilst advocating for that child and family when they need you to. You need to be able to connect with children of all ages and backgrounds, and be able to have fun whilst remaining professional. You need to understand that you are caring for the future population, and that the health choices they adopt now form the basis of their future and the generations to come.

References

Advanced Life Support Group (2011) *Advanced Paediatric Life Support: The Practical Approach*, 5th Edn. West Sussex: Wiley-Blackwell.

Bretherton, I. (1992) The origins of attachment theory. In John Bowlby and Mary Ainsworth, *Developmental Psychology* 28(5): 759–775.

Davies, R. and Davies, A. (2011) *Children and Young People's Nursing Practice: Principles for Practice*. London: Hodder Arnold.

Department of Health (2004) *National Service Framework for Children, Young People and Maternity Services*. London: DH, www.dh.gov.uk/en/Publicationsandstatistics/Publications/Publications PolicyAndGuidance/DH_4089100 (accessed 3 March 2014).

Glasper, A. and Charles-Edwards, I. (2002) The child first and always: The registered children's nurse: The first 150 years. Part 1. *Paediatric Nursing* 14(4): 38–42.

Ministry of Health (1959) *The Welfare of Children in Hospital* (Platt Report). London: HMSO.

National Health Service (2012) *Children's Nursing: NHS Careers*. London: NHS, www.nhscareers. nhs.uk/explore-by-career/nursing/careers-in-nursing/childrens-nursing (accessed 5 March 2014).

Nursing and Midwifery Council (2010a) *Children's Nurses*. London: Nursing and Midwifery Council.

Nursing and Midwifery Council (2010b) *Standards for Pre-Registration Nursing Education*. London: Nursing and Midwifery Council.

Rushforth, K. (2008) Celebrating child health nursing. *Paediatric Nursing* 20(5): 20–21.

Siviter, B. (2013) *The Student Nurse Handbook: A Survival Guide*, 3rd Edn. Edinburgh: Bailliere Tindall.

Further reading

Glasper, A. and Richardson, J. (2006) *A Textbook of Children's and Young People's Nursing*. Edinburgh: Elsevier Churchill Livingstone.

Nightingale, F. and Skretkowicz, V. (1992) *Florence Nightingale's Notes on Nursing (Revised, with additions)*. London: Scutari Press (original work published in 1859).

Randall, D. and Hill, A. (2012) Consulting children and young people on what makes a good nurse. *Nursing Children and Young People* 24(3): 14–19.

Useful web links

The Bristol Royal Infirmary Inquiry (2001): http://webarchive.nationalarchives.gov.uk/200908111 43745, www.bristol-inquiry.org.uk/final_report/report/index.htm

The United Nations Convention on the Rights of the Child (1989): www.unicef.org.uk/UNICEFs-Work/Our-mission/UN-Convention

The Victoria Climbié Inquiry: Report of an Inquiry by Lord Laming (2003): http://webarchive. nationalarchives.gov.uk/20130401151715, www.education.gov.uk/publications/eOrderingDownload/ CM-5730PDF.pdf

Life as a Children's Student Nurse: www.youtube.com/watch?v–wMH11Q8KwY

The history of nursing and midwifery registration: www.nmc-uk.org/about-us/the-history-of-nursing-and-midwifery-regulation.

Chapter 6

The uniqueness of mental health nursing

Catharine Jenkins and Cathy Poole

Mental health nursing is not a career taken up easily. Even by opening this chapter and beginning to read it, perhaps you are demonstrating an unusually open mind and willingness to look behind the stigma to explore how people in distress can be assisted by others. Perhaps you are wondering whether you could do this. I (Catharine) am an experienced mental health nurse and educator, and I would like to welcome you to this chapter, in which we will try to explain what our profession involves and why we find it so rewarding. Cathy's contribution to this chapter is to provide you with an insight into an alternative entry route into mental health nursing. Our aim is to clarify whether it fits with your motivations and could be a meaningful career choice for you. Terry McLeod explains how he got into mental health nursing:

> I never had doubts about dedicating my professional life to nursing, which I loved. Initially I started as a general nurse, and after a few years I moved to mental health nursing. I soon discovered this was my place. People suffering from mental health problems can feel very vulnerable, stigmatised, lost and hopeless, so there was plenty of work to do. Training was challenging: learning to establish good therapeutic relationships with patients and their families, bringing empathy, encouragement, and hope to their lives. Can you find something more rewarding than this?
>
> Terry McLeod BSc Nursing (Mental Health)

The job of mental health nurses is to work with people with a wide variety of problems affecting their ability to cope with life, relate to others or feel safe and in control. When put like that, it is clear that all of us have difficulties in these areas occasionally. This reflects our belief that mental illness is not something that 'happens to other people' – it can happen to anyone, and recent statistics indicate that it probably will (DH 2011). There is a stigma attached to emotional distress and partly for that reason we have chosen to refer to people who use mental health services as 'service users'. The title 'patient' seems to imply waiting for expert attention while 'client' is rather consumer-oriented. This leads us to one of the central characteristics of mental health nursing, which is that we can make a discussion out of anything – nothing is taken for granted and ideas are developing all the time. Similarly, because no two people are the same, regardless of diagnosis or professional experience, a career in mental health nursing will be one that is always fresh and interesting. So within the first couple of paragraphs you have probably already realised that mental health nursing attracts a different type of recruit! Service users are individuals with all sorts of family, cultural, social and economic backgrounds, so we need mental health nurses that reflect that diversity.

Some students from Birmingham City University illustrate this:

> I became a nursing student aged 54. My early education had been traumatic but I didn't understand why. Dyslexia wasn't then recognised, and the priority was being able to write clearly and spell properly – without those skills understanding and enthusiasm had little value. I did the classic 'drop out' thing, inner-city bedsits and grotty factory jobs, before being rescued by the Metropolitan Police (strange but true). Policing allowed me to develop at my own pace – they don't expect you to manage a murder enquiry from day one! I had an interesting and varied career. Spending cuts made it likely that I would be required to retire early, so I signed on as a mental health student nurse. It was a brilliant decision – I would recommend this career to anyone who really cares about other people. So, if you're an older student, or have so-called 'learning difficulties', just go for it! The training supports your own development and will give you the skills to enable others to achieve fulfilment.
>
> John Beddows BSc Nursing (Mental Health)

> After I had graduated with a degree in history from university, I worked in various support worker roles; working with young adults and people living with HIV. I realised that not only did I want to help people in similar situations, but I had a real interest in listening to people and wanting to get them to a 'better place'. Studying to become a mental health nurse has given me the opportunity to work with a wide range of people from various settings, who are all individual in their approach, needs and wants. It has challenged my beliefs and helped me to learn more about myself as a person. My .confidence in communicating with others in a variety of ways has also increased. My favourite aspect of the course so far is that the issues around mental health continue to surprise me. Being on placement for the first time was such a rewarding experience and really highlighted the important role a mental health nurse plays.
>
> Ellen Fielding BSc Nursing (Mental Health)

Certain personal characteristics are particularly useful. A compassionate, thoughtful and accepting approach to other people is essential, as is an intention to learn from and support service users and colleagues throughout your career.

The aim of mental health nursing is to work with individuals and communities to promote well-being, particularly emotional well-being, as a component of health. The idea of mental health differs according to the priorities of each person, but we could probably agree that it includes the capacities to enjoy ourselves, bounce back from troubles, get on with other people, and organise and manage our lives. In structuring our work to achieve this, we are guided by government policies, a code of conduct (NMC 2008), feedback from service users and a values and evidence base.

Foundations of mental health nursing

The history of mental health nursing is a fascinating subject. Originally people who looked after the mentally ill were called lunatic or asylum attendants, but eventually by 1912 we became 'psychiatric nurses'. While the emphasis of the care provided was on the mentally ill and often consisted of carrying out psychiatrists' wishes, following the Butterworth Report (DH 1994) it was agreed that we would be called 'mental health nurses'. This reflects an increasing emphasis on mental health and health promotion rather than illness, together with a focus on the importance of the therapeutic relationship between the nurse and those seeking care. If you would like to learn more about this, we recommend that you look at the work of Peter Nolan (1993).

Positive working relationships are essential to all fields of nursing. Service users need nurses to work with them towards their goals. Mental health nursing goes further than other fields of nursing because the therapeutic relationship not only underpins everything we do – it is also the main resource that allows us to achieve our aims. Mental health nurses need to establish positive professional relationships with people whose ability to form relationships is often disrupted by feelings of anxiety, low mood, confusion or fear. The people we serve may also have had previous experiences where others have not helped or have even been abusive or undermining. People may feel wary of us, they may have concerns about the stigmatising labels sometimes associated with mental health services, or feel that they would prefer not to risk trusting another person. This means that mental health nurses need to develop a sense of self that allows others to feel safe and optimistic, and then convey this effectively. They also need to listen attentively to people's concerns, showing interest, concern, empathy and a positive respectful attitude. This is essential because the care we offer has its foundations in the relationships we build.

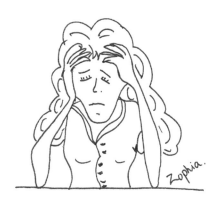

Each of us is unique, whatever our role or whether we feel mentally well or emotionally stressed. Our approach is based on respect for ourselves and others as people who respond to life's challenges sometimes with resilience and humour, sometimes with despair or fear, but most of the time somewhere in the middle. We accept that it is part of being human to have difficult times, and so we respond with compassion, genuineness and respect in the interactions that strengthen the relationships upon which mental health nursing depends.

Mental health nurses work with people from every background, of all ages, all ethnic, cultural and religious groups, all abilities, sexual orientations and social groups. We also work with people with a diverse range of problems, including: phobias, anxiety, obsessive compulsive disorder, depression, bi-polar disorder, schizophrenia, dementia, personality disorders, eating disorders, drug and/or alcohol addiction issues, post-traumatic stress disorder and postnatal depression. These problems can lead people to feel very strong emotions, such as sadness, loneliness, fear, frustration and desperation – sometimes to the extent that they act upon suicidal thoughts, self-harm or become temporarily unable to look after themselves and manage their lives.

People do not come into mental health nursing ready-made to take on these challenges. In fact, qualified mental health nurses will admit to constantly learning more about themselves and the skills they use. As a starting point it is important to accept that we are all potentially vulnerable and all potentially resilient, and that it is possible to learn how to look after our own mental health, and then use this understanding as part of our approach to supporting others.

The nurse and service user can be innovative in developing ways of working – perhaps focusing on an activity that has meaning that raises self-esteem and aids recovery. This activity may be different for each person, but whatever it is, the service user is likely to feel encouraged and supported by the nurse. Some people may prefer to talk one to one, or interact while taking part in sport, art, music, writing, gardening, cooking or walking. For some people, the most important thing the nurse can do is to keep them safe until they are able to do this independently again. Each individual will have their own path to recovery, using the relationship with the nurse to reconnect their own physical, emotional and spiritual health and their ability to be both part of a community and function independently.

In considering the goals of their work, nurses need to get to know each person, show empathy with their feelings and plan how they will work together to achieve the person's aims. For some people, their idea of what mental health looks like for them will be specific. Perhaps they will want to be back at work, getting on well with family and friends. Other people may not have such clear ideas and may be focused more on having relief from anxiety or whatever the problem is that brought them to mental health services. Some people may want to address the problem using medication, while others would rather try any other method first. It seems that 'mental health' is very individual and difficult to define. While some people might think that mental health is the opposite of mental illness, we would suggest that it is more than this, and while it varies from one person to the next, it always encompasses the ability to develop strategies to cope with life, to make relationships with others and to feel oneself to be a valuable person.

Many people struggle with issues that have a big impact on their feelings but are outside their control. For example, living in an area of high unemployment, where the environment is polluted, noisy and potentially dangerous might lead a person to feel anxious or depressed. The number of people affected by such mental health problems is surprising. The statistic 'one in four' is mentioned in health promotion, anti-stigma campaigns and government policy (MIND and Rethink 2008; DH 2011), but this does not tell the whole story. It is not one in any four! Oppression, poverty and diffi-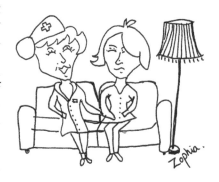cult life experiences, particularly in childhood, make people more vulnerable to mental health problems later on. One of the qualities of mental health nurses that other professionals respect is the ability to be with people who have experienced very challenging and distressing times. Most people believe they would be overwhelmed with sadness, sympathy or fear, but the mental health nurse is the one who is there to listen and to accept the person and their story. A recently qualified nurse explains her initial worries:

One thing that I found personally challenging during my first few months as a student nurse was the fear about my ability (or lack of it) to work with people who had a mental illness. This was mainly due to the stigma attached to mental illness. However, this 'fear' slowly lifted the more I gained insight and knowledge into the area, and certainly by the end of my first year I was much more comfortable and eager to go out on clinical placements and get involved in patient care.

Hadjer Bensiali, newly qualified mental health nurse

Being with people may not be easy, but is hugely valued by service users who may be otherwise rejected or not believed. To do this, mental health nurses need to accept their own feelings, manage emotions and listen to and support each other. The team the nurse works with is a great source of strength and experience and allows each member to grow and develop the skills and strengths required for this challenging, often invisible but professionally unique aspect of the role.

The connection between social and environmental factors and the impact on emotional health means that the role of the mental health nurse is increasingly widening to include interventions that address these root causes. The nurse does not only focus on individual distress but also increasingly on family and community well-being. Family-oriented work includes family therapy, initiatives that support social inclusion, and education about all aspects of health. Health-promotion work at a community level can involve educational initiatives, development of online resources, local community events or even theatre, often delivered through partnership working with service users, other professionals and voluntary groups.

Mental health nurses face a number of challenges in their roles. There is a stigma attached to mental illness and people in emotional distress and often their families too can find it difficult to approach services for help. Without care and treatment some mental health problems can worsen, leaving the person at risk of self-neglect, self-harm or other risky behaviour, including suicide attempts. Some aspects of mental illness, for example hearing voices, can be very frightening for the person experiencing them, who may react angrily or defensively, using possibly threatening language or behaviour. Alternatively, the person may withdraw from others so as to keep themselves feeling safe, or they may feel the need for constant reassurance to assist with coping with a feeling of agitation or anxiety. Mental health professionals, particularly nurses who spend the most time with people in distress and develop the closest relationships with them, need to manage these challenges in a way that keeps everyone involved safe, maintains each person's control over their life as far as possible, generates hope and then enables the person to rebuild their life and gain strength through the experience.

The nurse also needs the skills to provide sensitive boundaries, to assist in maintaining good physical health through nutrition, exercise and sleep, and to monitor responses to medication. The nurse needs the ability to keep calm in moments of tension, to recognise the emotion behind behaviour and respond in a way that protects the person's dignity. The interventions that mental health nurses use are based on core values taken from the work of Carl Rogers (1902–1987). Rogers was a psychologist and the originator of the person-centred approach to counselling. He suggested that the core conditions of empathy, genuineness and unconditional positive regard underpinned all therapeutic interactions and were essential in the process of a person achieving their own potential (Rogers 1951). The humanistic values promoted by Rogers are the basis of the nurse's need to show compassion, protect the dignity of those in their care and show respect for each individual.

The concept of 'recovery' has grown from the experiences of people with mental health problems themselves (Coleman 1999; Romme *et al.* 2009). Within this model the experts are not psychologists, nurses or theorists, but instead are people with histories and current experiences of depression, psychosis, anxiety and bipolar disorder. Not everyone who has a mental illness returns to how they were previously. That might not be possible, partly because of the intensity and life-changing nature of the experience and partly because some people's conditions and symptoms persist to some extent. The 'recovery' movement recognises that each person's journey and experience is unique, and it has a central concept of valuing the individual's perspective about what is meaningful for them and how they want their life to develop. The proponents, who are both service users and mental health workers, promote social inclusion and challenge the stigma of mental illness. The role of the nurse within this approach is to be open to the change that the service user identifies, then to work together optimistically as the service user reclaims their life (Barker 2009).

Service users also contribute to nurse education, as our colleague Colin identifies:

> I first came to the University in 2004, and all that was required of me was to tell my story, answer a few questions and go. Over the years, this has grown, along with my own confidence and abilities, from telling my story, helping co-facilitate classes, to taking lectures on my own, helping design courses to finally culminating in obtaining my postgraduate certificate in education and helping deliver a course to nurses on their final placement. It is a requirement that service users are involved in the educational process, but I feel that it is no longer an exercise that service users are there to tick a box, but academics have realised the depth, knowledge and substance they can add to the educational process.
>
> Colin Burbridge, mental health service user

Mental health nursing is influenced by several factors (see Figure 6.1). It is guided by three very specific theoretical perspectives. First, the interpersonal tradition (with emphasis on the nurse–patient relationship) based on Hildegard Peplau's (1952) work and developed in the UK by Professor Phil Barker (2009); secondly, evidence-based (what has been proven to work) mental health care, developed in the UK by Professor Kevin Gournay (1999); and thirdly, the recovery model, discussed above, based on mental health service users' own perspectives (Norman and Ryrie 2009). We are, however, also significantly influenced by the Department of Health, which in turn is influenced by the government of the day. Mental illness is one of the most expensive long-term and chronic conditions in the UK, so a large proportion of policy is seeking to reduce the impact on the economy as well as on individuals and communities. If you are considering mental health nursing it is useful and fascinating to follow policy development because it is such an important determinant of your chosen area of work.

Clinical knowledge, theoretical understanding, clear values and a strong evidence base are pivotal to the nurse's development. Sometimes it can be hard to tie it all together though, and this is where reflective practice comes in.

Mental health nursing is full of dilemmas. For example, when working with an older lady with dementia, she may ask you if she can now go home to her mother. It is hard to know what to say. The code of conduct (NMC 2008) directs us to be open and honest, so some people would advocate telling the truth, which might be that sadly her mother has died and she now lives in this nursing home. Others might suggest that as we make the care of people our first concern, a kindly fib would be appropriate. A student nurse who has read about Kitwood's (1997) ideas might recognise that the lady is indicating that she feels a need to be comforted or for attachment to others, so she could respond with, 'I'm sorry, your mum isn't here, but you're with me and I'm going to make sure you're all right. Shall we go together and see if the cat's in the garden?' The lady herself may not be able to articulate the sense that her dignity has been protected, but later on the student might reflect on what

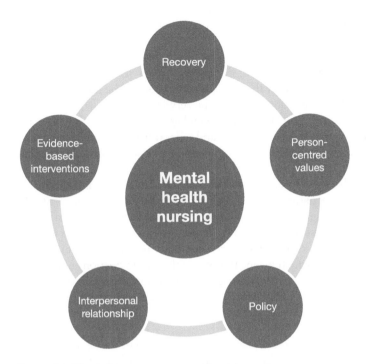

Figure 6.1 The influences on mental health nursing

happened and whether she should say something similar when this happens again. She may not know it, but another nurse who observed the incident may also be reflecting, and in the light of this decide to alter her own approach. The outcome of reflection should be greater self-awareness, sensitivity to the perspectives of others and, importantly, a change in practice.

Putting theory into practice

Mental health nurses practise in a variety of locations. The care we offer is increasingly community-based, although many work in hospital environments. Community work usually involves visiting service users in their own homes to offer interventions where people feel more comfortable, where they have the ongoing support of their family and where the structure of their lifestyle will not be disrupted. If the person needs more intensive support then their care will be provided through an in-patient admission. Following the closure of most old-fashioned large hospitals, care nowadays tends to be provided in smaller specialist units. Here care and therapeutic interventions are supplemented by opportunities for keeping fit and for learning or maintaining skills. After qualification, most nurses specialise and the profession offers many alternatives to support this. So, for example, you could choose to work in acute care, rehabilitation, with people with eating disorders, people who are homeless, with children and adolescents, or in dementia care, substance abuse or forensics. There is increasing awareness of the need for attention to the mental health of patients in general hospitals and as a result new liaison roles have been developed.

These specialist nurses offer advice and brief interventions, and are able to direct patients to other sources of support and information, often making use of Signpost UK (www.signpostuk.org/mental-health-issues).

Healthcare professionals are all team workers. Each profession has its own area of expertise and relevant skills. The multi-disciplinary team involves several different specialists organising together to meet the needs of service users. The relationship between the team members and their relationship with the service users and family members are crucial to achieving a positive outcome. Family members often have a caring role and can find this very stressful, so they need recognition and support from the professional members of the team. The team relies on feedback from the service user and family carers in planning their next steps.

Sometimes the feedback we receive indicates that the service user and the team have conflicting ideas about the nature of the person's problems. People with mental health problems do not always recognise that they need help and can become angry and aggressive towards mental health professionals, including nurses. At times we have to treat people against their wishes, in which case we have a responsibility to use the Mental Health Act 1983 (revised 2007) (MHA) which means that we apply certain Sections of the MHA to restrict a person in order to treat them. Treating a person against their will while remaining true to our person-centred philosophy can be difficult. Once again we return to how we develop a relationship with the person, so that they can learn to trust us and work effectively with the team for their recovery.

Like all nurses, we assess service users, plan their care, implement the plan and evaluate its outcome, then consider how we need to adjust the plan in the service user's best interests. Ideally all of this nursing 'process' should be undertaken in partnership with the service user, and with their wishes firmly at the forefront. The nurse will often take on a role of advocating for people when they are unable to articulate their wishes independently. At times the person will benefit from an independent advocate who will work with the team as directed by the service user. Occupational therapists, psychologists, social workers, physiotherapists, dieticians and many others liaise with nurses to provide the best interventions for service users. The nurse works together with medical and pharmacy staff over prescription of medication and then has the role of supporting the service user in getting the best from their input. These aspects of the role are essential for recovery, but are not all that the nurse does. Nursing is also driven by an evidence base, where research is used to ensure that effective interventions are offered. These interventions include therapies such as cognitive behavioural therapy, person-centred care, family therapy and anxiety-management strategies.

Entry into mental health nursing via the Army

There is an option to become a mental health nurse via the Army. This is known as 'defence nursing'. This route allows you to join the Army and complete a 14-week Phase 1 military training at Pirbright or Winchester where you will gain basic soldiering skills and fitness. Then you will be able to start your mental health student nurse training. Your undergraduate nurse training will be undertaken at Birmingham City University with civilian student nurses, and you will gain a BSc in Nursing. The three-year course is a mix of theory and practice, as defined by the Nursing and Midwifery Council (2010). Luckily you will be paid while you study. More details on Army pay can be found at www.army.mod.uk/join/25652.aspx.

When you qualify as a Registered Mental Health Nurse you will have the opportunity to travel and work overseas in MoD Hospital Units, Medical Centres or Medical Regiments. Wherever the Army is across the globe, mental health nurses are always required to meet the nursing needs of injured persons, maintain their health and prevent illness. As a nurse in the Army you will be part of the Queen Alexandra's Royal Army Nursing Corp (QARANC). Mental Health is provided through an extensive Defence Centre for Mental Health (DCMH) providing mental health support and advice facilities for service personnel, reservists, veterans and service families. Further information about becoming a mental health nurse via the Army can be found at www.army.mod.uk/rolefinder/role/228/student-nurse.

Conclusion

A person considering a career in mental health nursing is a courageous person. Not because the job requires bravery, but because it is emotionally demanding. The role is inspiring but it is not expected that a nursing recruit would have all the abilities described earlier, nor would all potential recruits be the same as each other – just the opposite! Service users are all different, unique individuals and come from a diverse range of backgrounds, and that is what nurses should be like too. Mental health nurses thrive in teams where they complement each other's strengths and support each other in developing their skills. Some nurses find they are naturally able to show endless patience with a person who is confused and distressed, while others need to learn the skill of communicating and connecting with someone who is losing their language ability and is feeling frightened and vulnerable. Similarly, some will find they quickly pick up how to give an injection, while another person will be practising in the simulation room many, many times. A potential mental health nurse will have some insight into the role for which they apply, will be able to give examples of times when the qualities described above have been demonstrated and will be determined to apply themselves to the demands of the nurse education course. Some people are drawn to nursing because of personal values, while others realise that their own personal skills 'fit' with the needs of nursing. Verona Reid is a qualified mental health nurse with many years' experience:

> My values originated from growing up in a culture where respect, caring and compassion were shown to others, especially the elderly; therefore nursing was my chosen profession even from a very young age. I can remember reading about the work of Florence Nightingale and Mary Seacole, their love and dedication for helping the sick, and this influenced my decision to be a nurse.

If you decide to go ahead and apply for a place on a mental health nursing course and are accepted, you will find that the course is structured to enable you to build your own understanding of what mental health is, what it means for you and what it means for others. You will learn how to protect and improve your own mental health through theoretical understanding and by interactive and reflective learning. You will be challenged in supportive environments, by staff with many years' experience who are there to help you thrive in your chosen profession. Your learning will be a process in which you take an active part, in which you support your peers and in return are supported by them. The course will be guided by current evidence and policy and will reflect service user feedback. You will find you learn more from service users than from your teachers – within the classroom, but even more so in practice.

Jodie Kirby is a 3rd year mental health student, about to qualify. She sums up her experience:

> During my training I have had a mix of challenges, experiences and opportunities that have helped me to develop my nursing skills. I have fundamentally changed my approach to nursing and now have a more holistic view. I have found many areas satisfying during my time as a student nurse. I have enjoyed gaining experience in speciality areas such as mother and baby services and the national deaf service for mental illness. What has kept me interested in mental health is the continually changing environments and learning new skills whilst overcoming challenges on a regular basis. I would recommend mental health nursing as it is a career that can progress in many different areas whilst continuing lifelong learning.

Mental health nurses find their job challenging but rewarding. It is a role for people who anticipate learning something new every day, who accept that there are not necessarily clear-cut answers to problems and who are willing to give more of themselves than in other professions. It is a role for people who are sensitive, caring and intelligent. It is a role for people who would like to feel they can make a difference to people's lives and in return make a difference to their own life. Terry McLeod, a Community Mental Health Nurse who recently retired, put it better than we can:

> I enjoyed all the training and development of the various roles along my career, but if you ask me to choose just one thing, I will tell you with no doubts, the best thing of all is the memories of the people I helped to recover. I do not think I could have found a more rewarding career, and if I had my time back, I know I would do it all again.

Mental health nurses need to be prepared to study, to reflect, to be compassionate, to be open, to find evidence, to challenge evidence and to use evidence. It is a role for people who are willing to work hard to gain the knowledge and skills required and combine them with their own caring qualities, for the good of others and for their own professional recognition and respect.

References

Barker, P. (2009) *Psychiatric and Mental Health Nursing: The Craft of Caring*, 2nd Edn. London: Edward Arnold.

Coleman, R. (1999) *Recovery: An Alien Concept*. Gloucester: Handsell.

Department of Health (2011) *No Health Without Mental Health*. London: DH.

Gournay, K. and Newell, R. (1999) *Mental Health Nursing: An Evidence-based Approach*. London: Churchill Livingstone.

Kitwood, T. (1997) *Dementia Reconsidered: The Person Comes First*. Buckingham: Open University Press.

Mental Health Act 2007. London: The Stationery Office.

MIND and RETHINK (2008) *Time to change*, www.time-to-change.org.uk (accessed 6 March 2014).

Ministry of Defence (2012) Defence Medical Services, www.gov.uk/defence-medical-services (accessed 10 October 2014).

Norman, I. and Ryrie, I. (2009) *The Art and Science of Mental Health Nursing: A Textbook of Principles and Practice*, 2nd Edn. Maidenhead: McGraw Hill/Open University Press.
Nursing and Midwifery Council (2008) *The Code: Standards of Conduct, Performance and Ethics for Nurses and Midwives*. London: Nursing and Midwifery Council.
Nursing and Midwifery Council (2010) *Standards for Pre-Registration Nursing Education*. London: Nursing and Midwifery Council.
Rogers, C. (1951) *Client-centred Therapy: Its Current Practice, Implications and Theory*. London: Constable.
Romme, M., Escher, S., Dillon, J., Corstens, D. and Morris, M. (2009) *Living with Voices: 50 Stories of Recovery*. Ross on Wye: PCCS Books.

Further reading

Brooker, D. (2007) *Person-centred Dementia Care*. London: Jessica Kingsley.
Nolan, P. (1993) *A History of Mental Health Nursing*. Cheltenham: Chapman & Hall.

Useful web link

Ministry of Health – Mental health support for the UK armed forces: www.gov.uk/mental-health-support-for-the-uk-armed-forces.

Chapter 7

The uniqueness of learning disability nursing

Fiona Rich and Marie O'Boyle-Duggan

Learning disability nursing is a field of nursing that has the same generic standards for competence as adult, child and mental health nursing, but also has unique field-specific standards for competence. Learning disability nursing is not like *ER*, *Casualty* or *Holby City* but that doesn't mean that the work we do is not critical or motivating.

What is learning disability nursing?

Many people are confused about what 'learning disability' means. Some people confuse it with learning difficulties – a term used for an individual who has a specific learning difficulty such as dyslexia. Others confuse learning disabilities with psychiatric or mental illness, which is a completely different field of nursing.

The confusion may lie in the fact that, historically, people with learning disabilities and mental illness were all classified under the same Act of Parliament – the Mental Deficiency Act, 1913 (Department of Health (DH) 1913). This act used derogatory terms such as 'idiots', 'imbeciles', 'feeble minded', and 'moral defectives', and all the people covered were nursed together in the same institution. Further confusion may have arisen due to the frequent changes in terminology used to identify learning-disabled people throughout the past hundred years. You may be familiar with terms such as 'mentally defective', 'mentally subnormal', 'mentally retarded', 'mentally handicapped', 'mentally impaired', 'cognitively impaired', 'intellectually disabled' and 'special needs' – all of which have been used to identify people with a learning disability. It is no wonder that the lay person could be confused as to what it means to have a learning disability.

So with all this confusion, what actually is a learning disability? If you look at the DH (2001: 14) document, *Valuing People*, learning disability is defined as:

- A significantly reduced ability to understand new or complex information, to learn new skills (impaired intelligence), with:
- A reduced ability to cope independently (impaired social functioning);
- Which started before, with a lasting effect on development.

Importantly, the DH (2001) document emphasises that the definition of learning disabilities encompasses people with a broad range of disabilities. This means that when you work with people who have learning disabilities you will encounter a wide spectrum of needs and abilities. At one end of the spectrum, you will meet people with profound, multiple learning disabilities (PMLD) who have very complex physical disabilities, sensory disabilities and severe learning disabilities, and require intensive support for all aspects of their day-to-day needs. At the other end of the spectrum, you will meet people who have very mild learning disabilities who, with minimal support from a community learning disability nurse, are able to live independently in the community. There are also many people with learning disabilities who fall between these two poles of the spectrum, and because of the range of abilities and needs that people with learning disability have, learning disability nurses work in a variety of settings. This could mean that, once qualified, you could work with:

- Child and adolescent mental health services (CAMHS) where you would specialise in providing help and treatment for children and young people with emotional, behavioural and mental health difficulties.
- Older adults with learning disabilities – as with the general population, more people with learning disabilities are living to an older age but tend to develop symptoms related to old age much earlier, e.g. cardio-vascular problems, dementia, Alzheimer's, etc.
- People who have a dual diagnosis of learning disabilities and a mental health problem – this is a combination of complex needs which requires specialist services.
- Health facilitation teams, liaising with hospitals, GP practices and clinics to ensure that people with learning disabilities have access to primary and secondary health services, receive appropriate treatment and have their health needs met.
- Specialist services working alongside other professionals to meet complex specialist needs such as epilepsy, challenging behaviour or forensic issues.
- Community learning disability teams, as a nurse with a 'case load', supporting families and/or carers and people with learning disabilities who live in the community.
- Medium secure forensic services or prisons, working with people who have learning disabilities who have committed offences.
- Short breaks/respite care services, supporting people with learning disabilities who have a wide range of health and social care needs whilst providing parents and carers with a short break.
- Community residential supported accommodation services, providing specialist support to people with learning disabilities, enabling them to live successfully within the community and to access community facilities.
- Day centre services, supporting people with learning disabilities in gaining work, leisure and social skills.

Each person with a learning disability is unique and because of this, wherever the care is being delivered the learning disability nurse will provide individualised, person-centred health care. Owing to the wide range of needs that people with learning disabilities have, the intensity of support needed by individuals varies enormously. Some people may be independent and living in a home on their own or with a partner. The nurse's role in this case is to support them to lead as independent a life as possible. Others might live in a semi-supported unit or sheltered accommodation, which requires a little more support. Others might need 24-hour care because of the degree of learning and/or physical disabilities they may have, or because they are a danger to themselves or others.

Key attributes of the learning disability nurse

As with all nurses, key attributes include having respect for the individual, treating the individual with dignity, and being caring, compassionate and considerate. People with learning disabilities may have problems with processing information and may not be able to respond quickly to questions. This can be frustrating for the untrained carer; therefore a key attribute in caring for people with learning disabilities is to have an abundance of patience and a holistic understanding of the person, which includes the way in which they communicate and how this impacts on their outward behaviour. For example some people are labelled as 'challenging' because they may behave in certain ways (e.g. they may hit out or hurt themselves), but this behaviour may well be an attempt to communicate a specific need, which the nurse needs to accurately interpret.

The learning disability nurse needs to have excellent communication and observational skills. All people are able to communicate in some ways, but some people have even more subtle ways of communicating than an outward display of behaviour described above – for example, it could be a slight nod of the head for yes or a blink, or a twitch of a finger. Learning disability nurses need to be very observant of the subtle ways in which people with learning disabilities communicate. It takes patience and time to develop an understanding of some of the communication abilities that people with learning disabilities have.

The learning disability nurse needs to be able to assess and understand the individual in a systematic way and use sensitive human interaction to interpret their specific needs and plan appropriate evidence-based care.

Learning disability nurses must also be aware of the importance of how their own verbal and non-verbal interactions can be interpreted by people with learning disabilities and the impact these interactions may have. A person with a learning disability might want to please the nurse and give answers that they think the nurse wants to hear rather than saying what they really think for fear of upsetting the nurse or getting into trouble. The nurse must be mindful of how questions are phrased as they can be 'leading' – for example, if a nurse says 'You are happy living here, aren't you?' this may lead to the service user agreeing with the question, even if they are not happy.

Patience is also needed when supporting a person with learning disabilities to develop new skills, as the process may need to be broken down into minute steps which take time for the individual to learn. Nevertheless once a skill is achieved, however small a step, this is a great accomplishment for the service user – and very rewarding for the nurse. For further information on generic knowledge and skills please refer to Part 3.

In addition to providing individualised, person-centred care, the role of the learning disability nurse covers a much wider remit – it also involves liaising with other professionals and working with family and carers in the wider community. Good communication skills and excellent team work are essential attributes of a learning disability nurse.

The nurse must be mindful that people with learning disabilities can experience discrimination and negative attitudes from people

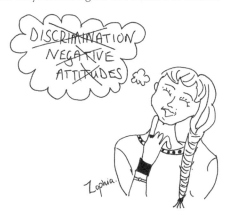

in society, but also from some healthcare providers. The nurse therefore must have a positive attitude, be assertive and project positive images of people with learning disabilities. At times this may involve challenging society's negative and discriminatory views.

Key themes studied

One of the major themes of learning disability nursing is the application of a person-centred approach to all aspects of nursing care, from assessing the individual's needs through to planning, implementing and evaluating care throughout the lifespan. This would include themes such as children with learning disabilities, adolescence, puberty, sexuality, parenting, the older adult and care of the dying.

The basic principle of a person-centred approach is to assist the individual (or those speaking on their behalf) to consider and express their own abilities, goals, and aspirations, and to plan how this might be achieved – it is not merely looking at the needs and deficiencies of the service user. This process also involves the individual's family and wider social networks. The person-centred approach therefore is not exclusively about what professionals identify as a need, nor does it mean that the individual's needs must fit in with the services currently available.

The easy-read version of *Valuing People* (DH 2002) defines person-centredness as:

> doing things in a way that the person wants and which helps them to be part of their community. If someone is in the centre of something, they are the most important person.

Communication is a theme that is essential throughout nurse training and is particularly important in learning disability nursing. Many people with learning disabilities have communication difficulties. They may have no verbal communication so they will need to use alternative methods to communicate their needs. This could be through the use of communication aids such as a picture board, by using objects or gestures to demonstrate what they are trying to communicate, or through the use of a simple sign language such as Makaton. Some people with learning disabilities who are unable to communicate their needs have learned that if they behave in a certain way, they will have their needs met, so use behaviours to communicate their needs. These behaviours can sometimes be seriously challenging and may involve self-injury, aggression towards others or damage to objects. In circumstances such as this it is important for the learning disability nurse to teach more appropriate methods to enable the individual to communicate their needs.

Some people with learning disabilities (and in particular people with autistic spectrum conditions) may not be able to interpret facial expressions and may become confused and anxious as a result. It is important for the nurse to be consistent with their use of facial expressions – and not, for example, frown when they are happy or smile when they are actually annoyed.

Another major theme of learning disability nursing, and one of the main roles of the learning disability nurse, is planning and implementing complex packages of care. This, hand-in-hand with person-centred planning, involves a holistic assessment of the individual and making a nursing diagnosis in order to determine the interventions required to meet their needs.

Nursing interventions for people with learning disabilities can be complex because there may be a number of clinical needs that must be met simultaneously. For example an individual may have Down syndrome with accompanying congenital heart problems, epilepsy, hypothyroidism and Alzheimer's disease (all of which are associated with people who have Down syndrome) but may also present with challenging behaviour. Care would be complex because one condition could be problematic for another condition – for example, hypothyroidism could accelerate the underlying heart problem present in Down syndrome.

People with learning disabilities generally have more health needs than those without, including heart conditions, problems with breathing, feeding/nutritional problems, diabetes, epilepsy, or mental health problems, to name but a few. It is important that symptoms of physical ill health are examined thoroughly and properly investigated and not merely attributed to the fact that the person has a learning disability – a problem known as 'diagnostic overshadowing'. For example when an individual displays challenging behaviour, it is important that the nurse does not automatically attribute this to their learning disability but must investigate the reasons for this behaviour carefully, because pain or illness may be the underlying cause of the behaviour and must be ruled out before attempting to plan interventions to reduce the challenging behaviour.

Reflection and critical thinking that questions and examines evidence-based nursing is essential to the development of complex packages of care, and the learning disability nurse must be able to research and determine best practice in order to produce care packages for people with learning disabilities with a range of needs, as detailed below.

Epilepsy

People with learning disabilities are far more likely to have epilepsy than those without learning disabilities. The more severe the disability, the more likely the individual is to have epilepsy. Diagnosing epilepsy can be a long process and involve a number of tests, so the nurse must be able to support the individual throughout the diagnostic process. This can be a challenging role, particularly if communication is a problem or if the individual finds changes to their routine very stressful.

One of the main tools used in diagnosing epilepsy is the eyewitness account, so the role of the nurse in caring for people with epilepsy often includes teaching family and carers how to recognise different seizure types. Accurate observations must be kept to establish the causes and triggers, so that the individual can be more in control of their epilepsy. 'Seizure diaries' are an essential monitoring tool to achieve this.

People who have epilepsy are likely to be prescribed anti-epileptic drugs, so they should be monitored for effectiveness of the drug and any side effects that may occur. Some drugs also require regular blood tests to avoid toxicity and to ensure that drug levels are maintained within a therapeutic range.

The package of care would also include teaching the family and carers the first aid treatment for epilepsy. However, there may be occasions where the seizure lasts longer than usual or the person goes from one seizure into another without gaining consciousness. In this case the package of care should include a protocol for rescue medicines and actions that must be taken in a medical emergency.

Challenging behaviour

The package of care for a person with challenging behaviour needs to consider why the behaviour is occurring, what is motivating the behaviour and what is reinforcing it.

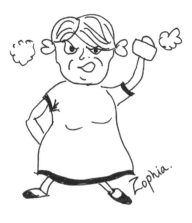

As previously stated, the nurse first needs to rule out ill health as a cause of the behaviour, so accurate assessments need to be carried out.

Positive-behaviour support approaches or interventions are considered within the themes of challenging behaviour and mental health, also referred to as a dual diagnosis. This involves a combination of systematic assessment and understanding of behaviours using applied behaviour analysis along with fundamental values such as rights, choice and inclusion, all set within a person-centred framework. The overall aim is that restrictive and punitive interventions are avoided and person-centred positive approaches of support are adopted

A person with challenging behaviour is likely to display behaviours that society finds unacceptable. These could range from unacceptable verbal behaviour or inappropriate attentions towards other individuals to aggressive behaviour, smearing faeces, or sexual behaviour such as public masturbation. The role of the nurse in these situations is to reduce the challenging behaviour by teaching more appropriate, socially valued ways of getting their needs met, with positive behaviour support.

Dual diagnosis

Statistically, people with learning disabilities are more likely to have mental ill health than the general population (RCN 2010). Life events that can affect all of us in terms of our mental health and well-being occur more frequently in people with learning disabilities. For instance, think of a time when you have moved house or left home, away from meaningful and significant friends – and remember how this affected you in terms of loss. Now imagine that you have a learning disability and that you have no understanding or control over this move – and no understanding of why your significant friends are no longer around. You can see how this can lead to extreme anxiety which often leads to depression.

A person with learning disabilities may experience changes to their environment for a number of reasons, causing a loss reaction. If you imagine a person with learning disabilities who is depressed through this type of loss, the likelihood is that this will go undetected. Carers may simply assume it is part of the learning disability rather than the underlying mental health issue. The role of the learning disability nurse is very important in assessing and understanding factors that can lead to a person with learning disabilities being mentally unwell, and they must plan and implement care that ensures protective factors are put into place. For instance, preparing a person sensitively for a move or meeting new staff in advance to reduce anxiety are protective factors (Bouras and Holt 2007).

Autistic spectrum conditions

Although autistic spectrum conditions are common in people with learning disabilities, they are often seen in people without learning disabilities (for example Asperger's syndrome).

The package of care for people who have learning disabilities and autistic spectrum conditions must address the fact that a person with autism may have particular characteristics that would mean they appear very remote and have difficulties in developing relationships. This can often lead to communication problems which can make developing relationships even harder, so alternative methods of communication should be considered.

A person with autism may have a very rigid routine which they have to follow each day, and if their routine is disrupted it could cause them a great deal of anxiety. The nurse needs to consider how any important unforeseen activities can be introduced to the individual without causing distress.

Complex physical needs and profound multiple learning disabilities

The package of care in this case must address the fact that the individual will have severe learning disabilities and little or no ability to self-care. They are likely to be completely dependent on carers to meet their personal needs, such as bathing, toileting and feeding.

This person will also have physical disabilities, meaning that they may have paralysis in their legs or arms (or both) as well as curvature of the spine or chest. Physical disabilities may mean that the individual has problems chewing and swallowing, so may need to be fed directly into the stomach through a tube (which can cause a risk of infection). Because of the inability to change position, pressure area care must be addressed. Lack of movement might also cause fluid to build in the lungs, causing a risk of infection which must also be addressed. In addition, the package of care may need to address sensory disabilities – hearing or visual problems.

Older adults with learning disabilities

Like the rest of the population, many people with learning disability are living longer because of improvements in healthcare. People with specific conditions such as Down syndrome, epilepsy and cerebral palsy have slightly shorter life expectancies than other categories of people with learning disability, but they too are living longer. Issues relating to ageing are more complex in people with learning disability because they are more at risk of physical disorders and diseases such as musculoskeletal, respiratory and cardiovascular illnesses, sensory defects, cancer, diabetes and fractures.

Some conditions such as Down syndrome have an increased prevalence of vascular disease, hypothyroidism, Alzheimer's disease, dementia, senility, hearing problems and decreased visual acuity – all of which occur much earlier than in the general population and could be as early as the age of 30. This requires a complex package of care and specialist interventions.

Ethical, legal and socio-political considerations

Another important theme involves the examination and consideration of ethical, legal and socio-political influences within learning disability nursing and the impact these have on interventions made. A learning disability nurse must then apply ethical, legal and professional principles to all aspects of care. For example, an intervention might include the need to make a number of restrictions on the individual in order to protect them from harm. The nurse must consider the Mental Capacity Act 2005 and the Deprivation of Liberty Safeguards (DoLS) before implementing a care plan which deprives someone of their rights. The learning disability nurse will need to have a working knowledge of a number of documents such as the Mental Health Act 2007, Human Rights Act 1998, Equality Act 2010, *Valuing People* (2001), and the *Healthcare for All Report* (DH 2008), to name but a few.

Learning disability nurses need to be politically aware of the impact that social policy has on shaping values and attitudes of all healthcare professionals. They have a key role in influencing positive attitudes towards people with learning disabilities and indeed in developing policies and training across healthcare settings to highlight the health needs of people with learning disabilities. This role extends beyond learning disability services into mainstream healthcare, where advice and consultation is provided to other health professionals. This ensures that current legislation is implemented to support people with learning disabilities more appropriately in acute healthcare settings. A number of reports – for example Mencap's *Death by Indifference* (2007); *Healthcare for All* (DH 2008); *Death by Indifference: 74 Deaths and Counting* (Mencap 2012) – all highlight examples of poor nursing care provided to people with learning disabilities in hospitals, due to lack of knowledge and understanding across the professions which in reality contravenes the Equality Act (2010). Education of other healthcare professionals is therefore essential.

Putting theory into practice

Evidence-based nursing care is a fundamental theme throughout nursing courses. Service users of healthcare expect nurses to know what they are doing and why they are doing it, and they expect things to be done well. It is not always easy for the student nurse to make the link between what they learn academically at university and how this is then applied when working with service users with a learning disability. Evidence-based nursing is about pulling together all the knowledge and experience gained, with the aim of creating a positive impact on the service user and the nursing care provided.

In order to put theory into practice, students are required to attend clinical placements where their competence is assessed based on the Nursing and Midwifery Council's (2010) Standards for Care. The nature and type of student placements reflect the diverse service provision identified earlier. They include placements within the NHS, private, independent and voluntary sectors, prisons, specialist-supported living accommodation, in-patient assessment and treatment units, and in the community, where students access family homes.

Students are prepared for placement in a variety of ways in order to provide them with sufficient theory to inform their practice. Teaching is not just about sitting in a classroom, listening to lectures, it is also about experiencing a wide variety of learning opportunities – for example, workshops, seminars, student presentations and simulated exercises, amongst others.

Simulated exercises are particularly useful in enabling students to put theory into practice. They allow students to learn and demonstrate skills and to consider the options for care in a safe environment that is not detrimental to service users, before attending placement.

Simulation may be of a virtual nature, where online simulated scenarios are provided, encouraging students to reflect, problem-solve and make decisions regarding nursing interventions. Here, any mishaps or mistakes form part of the learning process. An example of this can be seen at: http://shareville.bcu.ac.uk/index.php?q=resource/elmwood-house-new.

Simulation may also be 'live', where expert role-players act out challenging scenarios that students are likely to face in placement and where students must respond to the unfolding circumstances, using evidence from the theory element of the course to inform their actions. Examples of live simulation could include managing challenging behaviour, epilepsy, teaching a skill, gaining consent, communication difficulties and many more challenging situations that students are likely to come across in practice.

Assessments are also a useful way of helping students put theory into practice. Using a variety of assessment techniques, such as essays, student presentations, poster presentations, vivas, exams and OSCEs (objective structured clinical examinations), students can apply theory to practice and incorporate specific case studies into their assessments.

What is it like being a learning disability nurse? Testimonials from newly qualified and student nurses

I qualified as a learning disability nurse two years ago. I was a mature student and enjoyed every minute of my experience as a student. I even gained the student practice award and was extremely pleased with myself. Armed with pride and enthusiasm, I secured my first post and was full of excitement for my new adventure.

I applied for three posts after qualifying, as interview techniques are not my strong point. I was lucky enough to be offered all three posts and was then in a position to choose. I decided on a post working with people who were diagnosed with autism and also display behaviour that was considered challenging. This was an area that I found interesting. I was able to learn about forensic issues and also mental health needs, a great way to develop my skills and knowledge, as well as putting my own newly acquired skills to use.

It wasn't easy, and I would be lying if I said it was everything I had imagined it to be. There were highs and lows, and still so much to learn. I had gained really good skills at university but the reality of working life and all that comes with it was still difficult to adjust to. I have on occasion found it hard to remain focused and true to my profession. There were times when I questioned practice and that of the establishment, including my own personal qualities I had prided myself on. There were many times I had to fight my corner, and I sometimes felt like a lone crusader. The most amazing thing was that every now and again I was able to make a difference, sometimes only a small one, but nevertheless a difference that made me proud of the profession I had chosen. When things got particularly tough there was always a fellow learning disability nurse who I had met along my journey that I could call upon for guidance and support.

I was recently asked by a service user 'You're not a general nurse are you?' I replied 'No I'm not', feeling a little anxious about what she was going to say next. I said 'Why do you ask?' The lady smiled and said 'You stand out from the rest.' I smiled back and took the comment as a compliment. It made my day.

Nicola Payne, Staff Nurse (qualified 2010 from Birmingham City University)

As a student learning disability nurse about to finish the three years of training, reality hits – causing mixed emotions. Being a learning disability student nurse has been at times testing of my mental and physical ability, and you may think at some point, 'Is it all worth it?' Looking back now I can guarantee that it has been. Being on placements gives you the chance to have a break from the theory work at university and apply this knowledge into practice. Practical placements are a great learning opportunity and give you the chance to experience different areas. As a student nurse, I have been on placements in the community, within residential homes/nursing homes, and within a forensic unit.

Learning disability nursing is a unique qualification. Not only does it teach you how to provide high quality nursing care, it also teaches you to become companionate towards others providing a person-centred approach to individuals. Learning disability nurses are there to help to improve and maintain the physical, psychological and mental well-being of the clients within their care. Not only are you able to provide stability and support to the clients, at times you may become a client's advocate, enabling them to live a fulfilling and rewarding quality of life.

Whilst studying to become an RNLD (registered nurse learning disability) I feel that the course has set me up to become flexible in adapting the way I communicate with clients. I also feel that I have learnt to have a great deal of patience with the clients, especially the ones who display challenging behaviours, as at times it can become stressful. In addition, I feel that the course has enabled me to work well within a multidisciplinary team, ensuring that the client is always the main focus of our care.

Following on from this, the career path that I have chosen to pursue is as an RNLD staff nurse within a forensic unit. Being on my final placements has really helped me to focus on the career path I want to take.

If you're anything like me, you got interested in learning disability nursing because you have a true passionate desire to help and support people.

Rachel Jeffries, 3rd year student nurse, Huddersfield University

Summary

The learning disability nurse is someone who is not only caring and compassionate, but someone who can be innovative, imaginative, positive and forward-thinking to ensure professional and evidence-based care is provided.

Being a learning disability nurse means that you provide nursing care for the individual holistically, thus promoting complete physical and mental well-being and helping individuals maximise their potential to participate in society as fully as possible.

Because of the range of complex needs that people with learning disabilities present with, nursing care is provided in a huge variety of environments, from the individual's own home to specialist clinics, to health facilitation teams, prisons and in-patient assessment and treatment units. This also means that as a learning disability nurse you are working alongside and liaising with a wide range of other professionals – for example, psychiatrists, psychologists, speech and language therapists, dieticians, dentists, physiotherapists, occupational therapists and social workers – all of whom contribute to the holistic care of a person with a learning disability.

Learning disability nursing is not for everyone, but once you have insight into the difficulties that this vulnerable group encounter, either because of their personal limitations or because of the negative attitudes of some people in society, then there is no going back – you either try it and leave soon after, or try it and stay for ever.

References

Bouras, N. and Holt, G. (2007) *Psychiatric and Behavioural Disorders in Intellectual and Developmental Disabilities*. Cambridge: Cambridge University Press.

Department of Health (2001) *Valuing People: A New Strategy for Learning Disability for the 21st Century*. London: HMSO.

Department of Health (2002) *Valuing People: A New Strategy for Learning Disability for the 21st Century: Planning with People: Towards Person-Centred Approaches, Accessible Guide*. London: HMSO.

Department of Health (2008) *Healthcare for All: Report of the Independent Inquiry into Accesses to Healthcare for People with Learning Disabilities*. London: HMSO.

Equality Act 2010. London: HMSO.

Human Rights Act 1998. London: HMSO.

Mencap (2007) *Death by Indifference*. London: Mencap.

Mencap (2012) *Death by Indifference: 74 Deaths and Counting: A Progress Report, 5 Years On*. London: Mencap.

Mental Capacity Act 2005. London: HMSO.

Mental Deficiency Act 1913. London: HMSO.

Mental Health Act 2007. London: HMSO.

Nursing and Midwifery Council (2010) *Standards for Pre-registration Nursing Education*. London: Nursing and Midwifery Council.

Royal College of Nursing (2010) *Mental Health Nursing of Adults with Learning Disabilities, RCN Guidance*. London: RCN.

Further reading

Atherton, H.L. and Crickmore, D.J. (2011) *Learning Disabilities: Toward Inclusion*, 6th Edn. London: Churchill Livingstone.

Baron-Cohen, S. (2008) *Autism and Asperger Syndrome (The Facts)*. Oxford: Oxford University Press.

Clark, L.L. and Griffiths, P. (2008) *Learning Disability and Other Intellectual Impairments: Meeting Needs Throughout Health Services*. Chichester: John Wiley.

Grant, G., Ramcharan, P., Flynn, M. and Richardson, M. (2010) *Learning Disability: A Life Cycle Approach*, 2nd Edn. Maidenhead: McGraw-Hill/Open University Press.

Keenan, M., Henderson, M., Kerr, K.P. and Dillenburger, K. (2006) *Applied Behaviour Analysis and Autism*. London: Jessica Kingsley.

Useful web links

National Autistic Society: www.autism.org.uk

Autism West Midlands: www.autismwestmidlands.org.uk

Down syndrome: www.down-syndrome.org/case-studies/2008/?page=1

Epilepsy: www.epilepsy.org.uk

Mencap: www.mencap.org.uk

NHS careers: www.nhscareers.nhs.uk/details/Default.aspx?Id=123

Challenging behaviour: www.challengingbehaviour.org.uk

Makaton: www.makaton.org

Shareville: http://shareville.bcu.ac.uk/index.php?q=resource/elmwood-house-new.

How to become a nurse

Part 3

How to become a nurse

Chapter 8

What skills and qualities are important?

Cathy Poole

For some, the notion of becoming a nurse goes back to childhood and I often have conversations with prospective student nurses who recount stories of dressing up as a nurse and having played doctors and nurses. For them, becoming a nurses appears to be a natural progression. For others it may be that a family member or friend knows someone in the nursing profession, and their enthusiasm, commitment and passion for nursing ignites them to take up nurse training. Whatever the reason for choosing nursing as a profession, and before you progress any further and make that all-important decision to apply, you should take a look at your personal qualities and consider 'Do I have what it takes?' This chapter will outline for you the skills, qualities and personal attributes considered by many as the essential ingredients required to become a registered nurse.

Skills and qualities

If you look in any nursing textbook you will quickly come to realise that there are a variety of what are often referred to as 'personal attributes' – qualities or skills you will need in order to become a professional registered nurse. Now clearly throughout your three years training these skills will be honed and refined, so the question you should ask yourself is 'Do I have the basic qualities to apply for and begin my nurse training?'

Let's take a closer look at what we often refer to as the 'key skills' needed. Snow (2012) outlines what she believes to be the ten most important skills/attributes and I have added some additional ones (see Box 8.1). Whilst this list is not exhaustive it provides an insight, and perhaps it will prompt you to consider if you have these skills.

A critical personal skill needed in abundance is the ability to communicate well. Easier said than done, you may think! When considering communication skills what we really mean is your ability to communicate effectively, using verbal, non-verbal and written skills in what I often refer to as the 'communication triangle' (Figure 8.1).

Being able to effectively communicate verbally also requires a cocktail of additional skills, for example:

- Face-to-face dialogue
- Telephone skills
- Listening skills
- Ability to persuade and negotiate
- Ability to speak clearly and concisely
- Confidence.

Box 8.1 Skills and attributes of a nurse

Communication	Well-informed
Compassion	Sense of humour
Empathy	Open-minded
Sympathy	Non-judgemental
Patience	Tough
Endurance	Resilient
Caring	Approachable
Thoughtful	Welcoming
Knowledgeable	

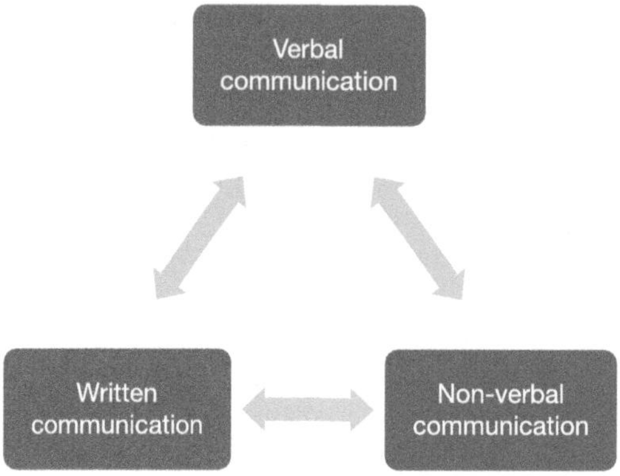

Figure 8.1 The communication triangle

Communication is not just about what is actually said – it is also about what language is used and how it is said, including the non-verbal messages transmitted through tone of voice, facial expressions, gestures and body language. It is often said that 'actions speak louder than words', reinforcing that body language is a powerful mode of communication. Body language can transmit both positive and negative messages, so being aware of your own body language is really important when dealing with patients, their families and, of course, colleagues.

When communicating information in the written form as a student nurse it is essential that a registered nurse countersigns on your behalf. The Nursing and Midwifery Council (NMC 2009) provide guidance on good record keeping. Some examples of this guidance are shown in Box 8.2. Full details of the guidance can be accessed via their website: www.nmc-uk.org/Documents/Guidance/nmcGuidanceRecordKeepingGuidancefor NursesandMidwives.pdf.

Hopefully this section on communication has made you think about your personal communication skills. Siviter (2004: 85) refers to the 'tools of the trade' (see Figure 8.2) in relationship to the skills that will be developed during your nurse training. You may already have these skills to some extent, depending on your previous experiences – but don't worry

---

Box 8.2 Examples of the NMC (2009) record keeping guidance

- Handwriting should be legible.
- All entries should be signed. In the case of written records, the person's name and job title should be printed alongside the first entry.
- Your records should be accurate and recorded in such a way that the meaning is clear. Records should be precise and clear.
- Records should be factual and not include unnecessary abbreviations, jargon, meaningless phrases or irrelevant speculation. Details of assessments, reviews, ongoing care and treatment must be recorded.
- You should use your professional judgement to decide what is relevant and what should be recorded. Records should be readable when photocopied or scanned.
- You must not alter or destroy any records without being authorised to do so.

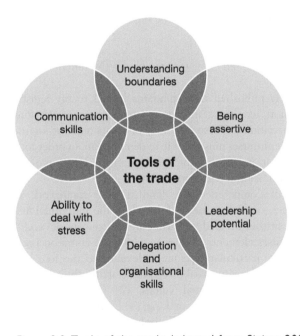

Figure 8.2 Tools of the trade (adapted from Siviter 2004: 85)

if you haven't, as these will be included during your training. The theoretical elements linked to these 'tools' will be taught whilst you are in the university setting and you will have ample opportunity to develop and practise them whilst on clinical placements throughout your three years training.

Whilst Snow (2012) and Siviter (2013) have outlined a selection of skills and attributes, I think that the ones they have listed are just the tip of the iceberg – and I can easily think of several more, such as:

- Having emotional stability
- Having stamina
- Being flexible
- Being resourceful
- Having the ability to pay attention to detail
- Having good interpersonal skills
- Having the ability to problem solve
- Having decision-making skills
- Being honest
- Being trustworthy
- Having respect.

With so many skills and attributes to consider, you may be curious to know what the NMC views are on the subject. One of the standards the NMC (2008) state is that professional nurses must:

Be open and honest, act with integrity and uphold the reputation of your profession.
(NMC 2008: 2)

Full details of these standards can be accessed via www.nmc-uk.org/Documents/Standards/The-code-A4-20100406.pdf.

The NMC (2010) have recently published new standards linked to pre-registration nursing education. This publication sets out standards of competence which must be attained during nurse training programmes. These standards of competence recognise the knowledge, skills and attitudes student nurses must be able to demonstrate in order for them to join the NMC professional register. For further information on the NMC professional register please see the section on professional regulation below.

The NMC (2010) standards of competence are detailed in a framework which consists of four sets of competencies, outlining one set for each of the individual fields of nursing. Each competence is then further divided into what are called 'generic' and 'field-specific' competencies. This recognises elements of nursing which are common (generic) and elements of nursing which have particular (specific) relevance to the four areas of nursing (adult, child, mental health, and learning disability). Additionally, the competencies are arranged into four domains: (1) Professional values; (2) Communication and interpersonal skills; (3) Nursing practice and decision making; (4) Leadership, management and team working. These four domains are undoubtedly linked to knowledge, skills and attitudes – so you can see how important it is for you to take a look at your skills and see how you can transfer them into your chosen career.

One additional fundamental skill that you will need is team working, which is linked to the NMC (2010) fourth domain. Nurses do not work in isolation but contribute to a health-care team, all of whom have the patients' best interests at heart. Therefore, from a team skills point of view you will need to have an understanding of how well you function as a team member. Before you can think about this, take a few minutes to consider who would

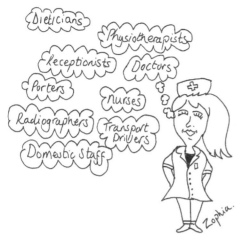

be in your team when working as a registered nurse. If you have a good understanding of the career you are about to embark on then I hope that you have quite a list of job roles which would constitute the healthcare team. For example you may have thought of the following: doctors, nurses, physiotherapists, porters, transport drivers, domestic staff, dieticians, receptionists and radiographers. This list is not exhaustive but serves to provide you with an idea of who you might be working with during your career. These team players are often referred to in the healthcare arena as the 'multi-disciplinary team' or MDT.

Much of the literature about successful team working relates to the role individuals play within a defined team. Miers and Pollard (2009) use terms such as 'co-ordinator', 'collaborator', 'team player', 'inter-professional' and 'multi-disciplinary team' synonymously when referring to the team approach to healthcare. Interestingly, they confirm that good team results rely on many of the attributes we have already discussed – for instance, communication skills, inter-professional relationships, personal qualities such as being punctual, being efficient and inspiring trust. Clearly, working with a variety of other professionals and non-professionals requires knowledge of those other roles, knowledge of when and how to include other members of the MDT, and therefore the ability to work across professional boundaries.

Recent evidence of poor quality care which has been highlighted in the media following the deaths of many NHS patients has raised the importance of care as a fundamental skill. This has culminated in the publication of the *Compassion in Practice* vision and strategy document (Department of Health 2012) drawn up by Jane Cummings, Chief Nurse for England. She has launched her vision based on six key principles, outlined as the six Cs:

1 Care
2 Compassion
3 Courage
4 Commitment
5 Competence
6 Communication

Clearly, these principles can be linked to the personal skills which, over the coming years, I am sure will become embedded in nurse training in terms of theory and practice.

Summary

Being a successful professional nurse requires you to have a vast array of personal skills and attributes, and nursing is certainly a complex career to be embarking upon. However, it can also be an extremely rewarding career, given the right personality. Certainly, the more of the traits above you have as an individual, the more likely nursing is the right career for you.

Whilst this chapter has mostly discussed the skills and attributes in general terms, of course there are also specialist skills you will need to consider, linked to the four branches of nursing. Further information on skills can be found in the relevant chapters (4–7).

Are there any other traits you believe nurses should have?

References

Department of Health (2012) *Compassion in Practice: Nursing, Midwifery and Care Staff: Our Vision and Strategy*. London: DH.

Miers, M. and Pollard, K. (2009) The role of nurses in the inter-professional health and social care teams. *Nursing Management* 15(9): 30–39.

Nursing and Midwifery Council (2008) *The Code: Standards of Conduct, Performance and Ethics for Nurses and Midwives*. London: Nursing and Midwifery Council.

Nursing and Midwifery Council (2009) *Record Keeping: Guidance for Nurses and Midwives*. London: Nursing and Midwifery Council.

Nursing and Midwifery Council (2010) *Standards for Pre-registration Nursing Education*. London: Nursing and Midwifery Council.

Siviter, B. (2004) *The Student Nurse Handbook: A Survival Guide*. Edinburgh: Bailliere Tindall.

Siviter, B. (2013) *The Student Nurse Handbook: A Survival Guide*, 3rd Edn. Edinburgh: Bailliere Tindall.

Snow, S. (2012) *Get into Nursing and Midwifery: A Guide to Application and Career Success*. Harlow: Pearson.

Further reading

Boyd, V. and McKendry, S. (2012) *Getting Ready for Your Nursing Degree: The StudySMART Guide to Learning at University*. Harlow: Pearson.

Crick, P., Perkinton, L. and Davies, F. (2014) Why do student nurses want to be nurses? *Nursing Times* 110(5): 12–15.

Elcock, K. (2012) *Getting into Nursing*. London: Sage.

Glasper, A. (2010) Widening participation in pre-registration nursing. *British Journal of Healthcare Assistants* 4(8): 391–393.

Useful web links

Nursing and Midwifery Council: www.nmc-uk.org/Documents/Guidance/nmcGuidanceRecordKeeping GuidanceforNursesandMidwives.pdf

Royal College of Nursing: www.rcn.org.uk.

Chapter 9

Applying for a nursing programme

Cathy Poole

Now that you have done your research on the different fields of nursing and decided which route you want to take, the next step towards your career choice is the formal university application process. This process can be confusing from the outset. You will have to become familiar with academic qualifications, tariffs, UCAS (Universities and Colleges Admissions Service) and its terminology, the timeframes, personal statements to support your application, the interview and selection processes, and the jargon linked to the offer and acceptance of places. This chapter has been written to help reduce the confusion and to help guide you through the application process. The UCAS website provides clear instructions and your current education establishment should also be encouraging and supportive in your application. A top tip therefore is to make full use of this help and also of the university websites.

Understanding academic entry requirements

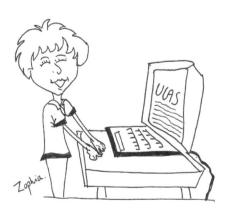

There are vast arrays of qualifications you can attain that will provide you with the academic entry requirements needed to secure a place on a nursing programme. For example, A Levels, BTECs, OCR Awards, Baccalaureates, CACHE Diplomas, 14–19 Diplomas or Access to Higher Education courses. You may even be eligible to apply to nursing as a postgraduate student if you have already gained a first degree. It is always worth studying the information on UCAS carefully, as well as the information supplied by the individual universities (in their prospectuses or online) to determine if you meet the required entry criteria. Despite the variety of qualifying courses you may find that a qualification you have is not listed on UCAS or the university website. Do not despair – contact the university admissions office (contact details are on UCAS and on the university websites). If the university admissions office is not able to help, they will put you through to the field-specific Admissions Tutor. Admissions Tutors are experts in their field and are familiar with the cocktail of courses students study today. They should therefore be able to answer your questions about entry qualifications.

Box 9.1 A level tariffs

A level grade	Tariff allocated
A*	140
A	120
B	100
C	80
D	60
E	40

Once you have established what qualifications are appropriate, you need to consider if you have them already or are working towards gaining them. Most universities will expect you to have already achieved the right level 2 qualifications, which are your GCSEs or their equivalent. The only exception to this is for those applicants who are undertaking access to higher education courses. All the universities which offer nursing programmes normally require applicants to have a minimum of 5 GCSEs (or equivalents in some instances) at grade C or above. They will also want your GCSEs to include English Language and Mathematics – and, more often than not, a Science.

So if you meet the level 2 requirements, you now need to consider if the level 3 subjects (A levels or their equivalents) you are studying are appropriate areas of study. Again the individual university websites and UCAS will list the subjects and, more importantly, the grades they are looking for in their applicants.

When looking at the level 3 requirements you will see that the different qualifications carry different 'tariffs', depending on grades. Box 9.1 shows you how this relates to A levels. Other qualifications have different tariffs for their various grades. UCAS provide a really useful tariff table which you can access at www.ucas.com/sites/default/files/tariff-tables-july-2012.pdf.

When you are looking at the tariff table you may discover that the level 3 qualifications you have or are studying for are not listed. Again, do not despair, as not all qualifications attract tariff points. So again it is worth contacting the universities which you are interested in, to see what their position is regarding your level 3 qualifications. If you have any questions about tariffs, UCAS are more than happy to help you – you can email your question to: tariffqueries@ucas.ac.uk.

How do tariff points relate to your university nursing application? Each university decides what total tariff applicants need in order to meet their entry criteria. They not only define the subjects therefore but also the tariff required. So do your research, as there is little point you spending time applying to a university only to find that your application is unsuccessful because of your tariff (or predicted tariff) or the subjects you are studying.

Navigating UCAS

When you first start looking at UCAS it can be quite daunting, so I think the first thing you need to do is to understand what subjects and their associated tariff you have by using the tariff link outlined above. Then you are in a strong position to begin to select the universities you are interested in. UCAS have produced a small video which explains how to navigate your way through the application process, so this would be a great place to start (www.ucas. com/how-it-all-works).

A lot of universities offer nursing programmes – but not all universities offer all four fields of nursing (and only Birmingham City University offers defence nursing). Your next step is to see which universities offer the programme of study you are interested in. Probably the easiest way to do this is to use the course search tool on UCAS (http://search.ucas.com). If you are not sure what part of the country you want to study in then you can do a broad search by entering 'England', 'Scotland', 'Wales' or 'Northern Ireland' and the search term 'nursing', and very quickly all the universities offering undergraduate nursing programmes will be listed alphabetically for you.

Now you are ready to review the course information on UCAS and begin to make some decisions about where you want to study. Box 9.2 shows some useful resources which will help you to decide which university to apply to.

Elcock (2012: 61–62) also provides useful advice on how to map the universities you are interested in. She suggests that you ask yourself several key questions relating to your university choice:

1   Which field of nursing do I want to study?
2   Which universities offer my field of choice?

Box 9.2 Resources to aid your university choice

Resource	Key content
Unistats and the National Student Survey	http://unistats.direct.gov.uk. This site allows you to view official government statistics on individual university outcomes in terms of students' satisfaction, student achievement and learning resources, for example.
The Student Room	www.thestudentroom.co.uk. This site boasts the largest student community in the world, offering advice on universities, health, accommodation and lifestyle, for example.
University league tables	www.thecompleteuniversityguide.co.uk/league-tables/ rankings?s=Nursing. This site provides information on university performance in terms of research, graduate careers, student to tutor ratio, and quality of teaching, for example.
UCAS	www.ucas.ac.uk. This site is pivotal to your research. It is informative for applicants, providing all key information and processes linked to your university application.
Individual university websites	All universities have online information about their courses and often have full prospectuses for you to download.

3   What do I want to get from my university of choice?
4   Where do I want to live whilst undertaking my nurse training?
5   If I do not want to move away from home, what universities are within my travel range?
6   If I move away from home, how often will I want to visit home?
7   Does the university of my choice have parking facilities?

Whatever questions you have, it is a good idea to create a spreadsheet of the answers you find during your research. That way, you will stay focused and make an informed decision when you finally press the apply button on UCAS. This mapping process will also help you to decide which universities you would like to visit prior to your final decision. There is nothing better than physically taking a look at the facilities and getting a feel for the place. This is explained in more detail below.

When your research is complete, it is time to complete your UCAS online application form. UCAS have an application flowchart for you to check out to make sure that you meet the application deadlines. It can be accessed via: www.ucas.com//sites/default/files/application-flowchart.pdf.

The most important thing to remember here is that if you miss the application deadline the universities are not duty bound to review your application, which may result in an early rejection. If you are still studying, your teachers/lecturers will be constantly reminding you about the application deadlines. Take note of their advice, as they want your application to be successful.

You can apply for five nursing courses in one UCAS cycle. You have to pay a fee, which is currently (2014) £12 for a single choice or £23 for two to five choices. If you use all five choices during the UCAS cycle you may be able to apply for more courses, using 'UCAS Extra', but only if you have received decisions from all five universities and you have not been accepted or you have decided to decline any offers you received. The current fee is £11 for each extra choice you make. UCAS have a great short video which clearly explains the extra application process. This can be viewed via www.ucas.com/how-it-all-works/undergraduate/tracking-your-application/adding-extra-choices. I usually advise students to use all five choices, as they may then find themselves in the luxurious position of having several offers!

In order for you to track your application and the progress made, UCAS requires you to register. Once registered you can easily track what is happening to your application form and, more importantly, see what offers the universities make you.

It is very important that you complete your application form fully and honestly. There are seven sections on the application form which you must complete:

1   Personal details
2   Additional information (for UK applicants only
3   Student finance arrangements (UK applicants only)
4   Course choices (up to five choices)
5   Education so far
6   Employment history
7   Personal statement.

Lastly, there is a reference section which needs to be completed by your referees. Again, UCAS provides very clear advice on how/who should complete this for you (see the short video at: www.ucas.com/how-it-all-works/undergraduate/filling-your-application/references-payment-and-sending).

Each section of your application form is critical, as it provides the basis on which your application will be assessed. I have often received incomplete application forms, application forms full of typing and grammatical errors, and even application forms where the personal statements make no reference to the field of nursing which the applicant has chosen to apply for. My best advice for you therefore is to get your application form thoroughly proofread before you apply. You must check, check and recheck before pressing submit. The section below on application selection criteria will give you some advice on what to include in your personal statement, as this is often an area of great anxiety for applicants.

University open days

All universities have open days. This is their opportunity to convince prospective students that their facilities, teaching and learning expertise, social activities, sports facilities and graduate career prospects, etc. are worth choosing – and will make an invaluable three-year contribution to students' lives.

You will be able to find out when individual university open days are by going onto their websites. In some instances you can register to attend in advance and even book times for the tours and talks which are scheduled throughout the day.

This is your opportunity to really make an informed choice about the university. You will be spending three years there and if you want to get a feel for the campus there is nothing better than meeting the academic teams face to face and having your questions answered. You will also meet people who are feeling as nervous as you about the prospect of going to university – it is undoubtedly a big step, especially for those of you who will be moving away from home for the first time. One of the key things you will want to know about is the accommodation facilities, so try and check them out. Prospective students often bring their parents with them – which is fine, because they are also likely to be anxious about where their children might be coming to.

On their open days, many universities have skills rooms set up as real wards (with manikins that breathe and have a pulse, surrounded by equipment which you commonly see in healthcare environments), so take every opportunity to see what this is all about. It is useful to have a very clear idea of what you are looking for in a university, and indeed the nursing programme, so you can tick off what they have or don't have. And you may find some things you weren't expecting.

Application selection criteria

There are several what I call 'sieving' stages you will progress through during the application and selection process:

- Qualification sieve
- Personal statement sieve
- Literacy sieve
- Numeracy sieve
- Interview sieve (one-to-one and/or group interview)

- Offer sieve (conditional/unconditional)
- Results day sieve.

Let us take a look at each of these individually, so that you are clear about what is expected.

Qualification sieve

It is paramount that you meet the entry criteria (often referred to as the 'entry profile') for whichever university you are applying for. It is vital that you include all your qualifications (level 2 and level 3). If you miss any off, your application form might be rejected by the university admissions officers and therefore not be sent to the admissions tutors for review. In this case, your UCAS track will indicate 'Unsuccessful Application'. You want to give yourself the best chance of your application form reaching the admissions tutor so get this right first.

Personal statement sieve

When your application form reaches the admissions tutors they will automatically check your qualifications and tariff (or predicted tariff) and they will then undertake a detailed review of your personal statement.

This is your opportunity to really explain why you have chosen to undertake the nursing programme and, more importantly, why you have chosen a particular field of nursing. Personal statements can make or break applications. Fergy (2012: 67) offers some really good advice on personal statements, which includes the following:

- Think and reflect long and hard about what you want to include about you
- Prepare a plan
- Seek advice and guidance
- Stick to the UCAS guidelines, i.e. no more than 4,000 characters and no more than 47 lines
- Draft your personal statement in Word first, using its spelling and grammar checks
- Be truthful
- Keep your focus.

When completing your personal statement, you need to consider which field of nursing you wish to apply for, e.g. adult, child, mental health, learning disabilities or defence nursing. Chapters 4–7 may help you decide which one you would like to learn more about. It is very important to be confident in your choice of field, as it is not always possible to change fields. If once you have started the programme you find that you do not like the one you have chosen, there may be the opportunity once on the programme to change fields, but this cannot always be guaranteed. When reviewing the universities, it is worth looking at the content of their programmes to establish whether you have to choose the field at the beginning of the programme or you can undertake a core first year, looking at all fields and then making your choice after having experience in all settings. When writing your personal statement ensure that you can clearly identify the field of nursing you are choosing and your reasons for doing so. If you have gained experience working in a caring setting, either as part of a college course or as work experience, make sure that you write about it. Talk about what you have learnt about the type of patients or service users you have nursed or worked with and your understanding of the profession itself, whilst working there. UCAS provide examples and top tips on how to complete the personal statement on their website – a really useful point of reference. You can view a short video about personal statements via: www.ucas.com/how-it-all-works/undergraduate/filling-your-application/your-personal-statement ?gclid=CIKQ7vH6vLwCFUjItAod418A0w. Most university websites also provide hints and tips on personal statements and it is a subject often raised by prospective students at university open days.

When reviewing application forms, the majority of universities will be looking for you to indicate that you have had some experience within a caring environment. Therefore it is really important that you do this – before you apply for a nursing programme. The reason you need to be confident of your career choice is that nursing is not as glamorous as it is portrayed in television series such as *Casualty* or *Holby City*. If you do not have any direct experience of caring, then the reality of nursing patients and service users when on placement may come as a shock.

One final piece of advice is make sure that your personal statement really reflects you. And make sure that you remember what you have written, as there is nothing more worrying for an admissions team during the interview process than having an applicant sitting before them who appears to bear no resemblance to the one who has written the personal statement!

Literacy sieve

The Nursing and Midwifery Council (2010) specifies literacy entrance requirements for all fields of undergraduate nursing – so literacy assessment must form part of the recruitment and selection criteria.

The selection criteria include evidence of a good command of both spoken and written English, which should include reading and comprehension. In Wales the same criteria apply to English or Welsh.

This requirement has seen the development of a variety of assessment methods used by individual universities as part of their selection and recruitment criteria. For example UCAS application forms are scrutinised and in some instances scoring criteria are used. Some universities have introduced written tests as part of their interview process which includes essay writing, paraphrasing, spelling tests, grammar testing or multiple-choice questions, for example. You will be able to find out what is required by looking on university websites. You may also find sample papers on some of the websites, and some universities outline literacy requirements as part of their open day information. Literacy assessment encompasses communication skills in both written and verbal forms, as well as information and communication technology (ICT) skills.

If you are from outside of the European Economic Area (EEA) and English is not your first language, the NMC (2010) require you to score at least 7.0 in the 'Listening and reading' and 'Writing and speaking' sections of the International English Language Testing System (IELTS). Additionally, the overall average IELTS score must be 7.0. So if you are a little rusty in this area and need some practice it is worth visiting the BBC Skillswise site for some practice via: www.bbc.co.uk/skillswise/English.

Being able to communicate clearly and accurately in nursing is a fundamental skill, which is pivotal to the safe, effective and uninterrupted delivery of healthcare, which is why so much emphasis is placed on these skills, not only during the recruitment process but also throughout the three-year nurse training programme.

Numeracy sieve

As well as literacy, the Nursing and Midwifery Council (2010) specifies numeracy entrance requirements for all fields of undergraduate nursing – so numeracy assessment must form part of the recruitment and selection criteria. The numeracy skills include:

- Addition
- Subtraction
- Division
- Multiplication
- Use of decimals
- Fractions and percentages.

The NMC (2010) further add that applicants must be able to use a calculator. So you must be prepared for your numeracy skills to be assessed during your application process. As with literacy, the universities have established a variety of methods for assessing numeracy skills, which mostly take place on interview days. The testing can be done using paper-based tests or electronically, using computer programmes which not only test your numeracy skills but also test your ability to navigate around a computer and follow instructions. These tests therefore have three purposes – this is numeracy, literacy and ICT testing, all rolled into one.

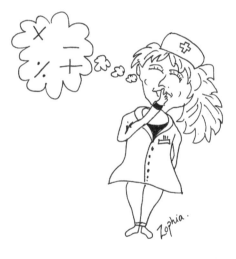

Elcock's *Getting into Nursing* (2012: 79–96) has some great examples of the type of numeracy test questions you will be faced with. You will also find example tests on some of the university websites.

Being able to confidently use what we call 'everyday maths' is an essential safety requirement in nursing. You will use your maths during medication administration, for calculating intravenous fluids, and measuring urine output, for example – which is why so much emphasis is placed on numeracy skills. So keep practising, and make sure you know what to expect with regards to individual university numeracy testing procedures. As the old saying goes, 'Failing to prepare is preparing to fail'.

Interview sieve

If you reach the interview stage you are now in a very good position to convince the interview teams that they should offer you a place to undertake nurse training with them. All nursing programmes include an interview in some format or another as part of their selection process. Figure 9.1 gives an idea of what to expect. The format of

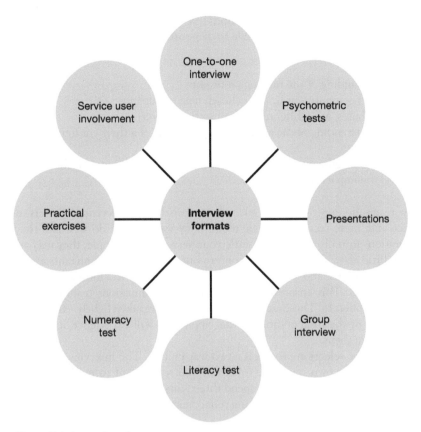

Figure 9.1 Interview formats

the interview is discussed at open days, advertised on university websites and often outlined in the letter inviting you to an interview, so there is no reason why any aspect of the interview should come to you as a surprise, as long as you have done your research. High on the NHS and NMC's agenda is patient engagement and service user views. This concept has been in many instances introduced into the selection process of pre-registration nursing students (Roberts *et al.* 2010). Therefore it would not be unusual for lay people to be part of an interview panel, and in some cases I have seen the introduction of information technology to engage participation of children and young people in this process.

An interview for a nursing course is often the first time that applicants have ever been interviewed, so this can be a really worrying time and can be the cause of great anxiety. So seek help and advice from your school/college or careers services and make absolutely sure you know what to expect on the day. It is really difficult to try and prepare you for all eventualities in this short section, so my best advice is to ask for help. Schools and colleges often arrange mock interviews and I would recommend that you participate, if you can. The Student Room offers some helpful tips which you can access via: www.thestudentroom.co.uk/wiki/nursing_interviews.

Snow (2012) offers a comprehensive range of really good advice, including an interview survival kit. No matter what format the interview takes, the selection teams are really trying to establish if the candidates are able to demonstrate the following knowledge and/ or potential:

- a sound understanding of the nursing profession;
- motivation and commitment to their chosen field of nursing;
- skills and attributes, as highlighted earlier in this chapter;
- a realistic understanding of the academic requirements of a three- or four-year nursing degree;
- appreciation of juggling personal time around the theory and practice challenges;
- understand the impact of shift work.

Interview teams are experienced people, often consisting of university lecturers, nurses from practice and, more recently, service users. They want you to do well and they will often use questions initially to help you settle your nerves – for example, they may ask you to tell them a little about yourself. During one-to-one interviews all applicants are usually asked the same questions, and a scoring matrix is used to mark the individual candidates using sample answers. This ensures parity, and helps the admissions team decide which candidates to make offers to. These are not decisions which are taken lightly – the admissions teams are mindful of the disappointment that applicants will experience if they do not receive an offer from them.

Remember that the selection process is a two-way process. The interview offers you the opportunity to ask your own questions – because you really want to make sure that this university is the one where you want to spend three years of your life. You asking questions also has the positive impact of demonstrating your commitment, enthusiasm and categorical desire to study with them.

You may find that some universities get applicants to undertake literacy and numeracy testing at the start of the interview process. Applicants who have achieved the pass mark will then progress to the next stage – face-to-face interviews, for example. Details of processes such as these will be explained in your invitation to an interview letters, at open days and on the university website.

Offer sieve

All universities who offer nursing programmes can only recruit to a certain number, as their nursing places are funded by Health Education England. There are usually more applicants for nursing programmes than there are places available – so competition for places is tough. Waiting to see if the universities make you an offer is extremely stressful. You will receive notification via your UCAS track. Some universities do not make any offers until they have interviewed all their prospective applicants – so what they are doing is making offers to the best candidates. This is why it is important to use your five choices from the outset to increase your chances of being made an offer. I know of many applicants who do not get an offer from any university when they first apply – but this does not deter them, as I have seen them return the following year, having gained some experience and learnt from their previous application process and taken steps to do better second time round.

Box 9.3 UCAS offer terminology

Conditional offer	Offer of a place which is dependent upon you meeting certain conditions.
Unconditional offer	Offer of a place on a course with no conditions – the place is yours to accept.
Firm choice	An offer you accept as your first choice, usually the university you like the most.
Insurance choice	An offer you accept as your second choice, usually with a lower tariff, as a back-up – just in case you fail to meet the conditions of your firm choice.
Deferral	If you want to take a gap year you can transfer your offer to the next academic year.

When the offers are made to applicants they will either be 'unconditional' or 'conditional'. If you already have the right level 2 and level 3 qualifications and meet the entry tariff you would be made an unconditional offer, because you meet the current criteria. If you are made a conditional offer, it is usually because you are still waiting for your level 3 qualification results, and particular conditions are therefore put on the offer. The details of your offers are explicit, and if on results day you do not get the specified grades or tariff your offer will not translate into a firm offer, and that place will be lost.

When an offer is made to you, you have to decide whether you want to accept it as your 'firm' choice or make it your 'insurance' choice. Box 9.3 outlines what the offer terminology means. UCAS has a list of terms with their explanations, which you may find helpful, at: www.ucas.com/ucas-terms-explained.

Fees and funding

Most students who attend university have to pay university fees. This is not so for students who choose nursing programmes, because their fees are paid for by Health Education England (HEE). HEE have a responsibility to advance the quality of care delivered to patients, which is achieved by placing focus on the education, training and development of current and future healthcare staff. HEE have 13 Local Education Training Boards (LETBs) to whom they delegate local responsibility for the commissioning of training and education of NHS staff. Therefore the majority of students who undertake courses in nursing which lead to registration with the Nursing and Midwifery Council are eligible for financial help from the NHS during their studies. This financial support usually extends to:

1 Payment of tuition fees
2 A non-means-tested bursary of £1,000 per year
3 A means-tested bursary.

Detailed information about your eligibility for an NHS student bursary can be found on the relevant country websites (see web links at the end of this chapter). You will find an online bursary calculator on the bursary website which is a very useful tool to give you an idea of the amount of funding you can expect.

When you start to explore NHS student bursaries you will see that there are some personal circumstances which will influence how much you will be entitled to, for example:

- Dependants' allowance
- Childcare allowance
- Parents' learning allowance
- Disabled students' allowance.

Given that 50 per cent of your three-year training programme is spent on clinical practice placements, consideration of the costs for this is recognised. The NHS therefore provide help with travel costs to your placements, as long as the cost is more than you would normally pay to travel to university, and providing you are eligible for the £1,000 grant.

When you have had an offer (conditional or unconditional) from a university you will be able to apply for your NHS Bursary and Grant online, through the Bursary online support system (BOSS) at: www.nhsbsa.nhs.uk/Students/4002.aspx.

You will also be able to apply for a reduced rate student loan from Student Finance England at: www.gov.uk/studentfinance. You can do this either before or after you have applied for your NHS bursary.

For mature students, often one of the biggest worries is the money side of being a student. But somehow their overriding determination to embark on a professional nursing career and their commitment to their chosen field of nursing gets them through their 'three years of austerity', enabling them to then embark on a career of a lifetime and a nursing world of opportunities.

Summary

This chapter has most likely given you a great deal to think about and reflect upon, but hopefully it has taken some of your anxiety away and has provided you with some clear guidance.

Your university application is a two-way process. You are choosing which programme at what university best suits you. The university, on the other hand, is choosing which applicants they want on their programme – those who come with the right entry criteria and are able to convince interview panels that they have the right cocktail of qualifications and personal traits which will make them suitable candidates to ultimately enter the nursing profession.

So good luck with your research and your application, and remember to seek advice throughout the process from the range of resources which are available. Importantly, if you are unsuccessful during your first round of applications this does not preclude you from reapplying during the next UCAS cycle. As the old saying goes, 'If at first you don't succeed – try, try again'.

References

Elcock, K. (2012) *Getting into Nursing*. London: Sage.

Fergy, S. (2012) *The Application Process and Choosing the Right University*. In Elcock, K., *Getting into Nursing*. London: Sage.

Nursing and Midwifery Council (2010) *Standards for Pre-registration Nursing Education*. London: Nursing and Midwifery Council.

Roberts, P., Wild, K., Washington, K., Mountford, C. and Priest, H. (2010) Inclusion of lay people in the pre-registration selection process. *Nursing Standard* 24(48): 42–47.

Snow, S. (2012) *Get into Nursing and Midwifery: A Guide to Application and Career Success*. Harlow: Pearson.

Further reading

Borrego, M. and Baird, J. (2010) *Careers Uncovered: Nursing and Midwifery*, 2nd Edn. Richmond: Trotman.

Boyd, V. and McKendry, S. (2012) *Getting Ready for Your Nursing Degree: The StudySMART Guide to Learning at University*. Harlow: Pearson.

Evered, A. (2013) *Get into Nursing School for Dummies*. Chichester: John Wiley.

Gatford, J.D. and Phillips, N.M. (2011) *Nursing Calculations*, 8th Edn. Edinburgh: Churchill Livingstone.

Shihab, P. (2010) *Numeracy in Nursing and Healthcare Plus MyMathLab*. Harlow: Pearson Education.

Useful web links

BBC Skillswise: www.bbc.co.uk/skillswise

NARIC (which provides information from as many as 180 countries in relation to vocational, academic, professional and skills qualifications): www.naric.org.uk

NHS bursaries

    for England: www.nhsbsa.nhs.uk/Students.aspx

    for Wales: www.wales.nhs.uk/sitesplus

    for Scotland: www.saas.gov.uk/_forms/funding_guide.pdf

    for Northern Ireland: www.nursingandmidwiferycareersni.com/bursary.html

English Language Testing System: www.ielts.org/default.aspx

Studential (sample nursing questions): www.studential.com/interviews/nursing-questions

UCAS

    home page: www.ucas.com

    tariff tables: www.ucas.com/sites/default/files/tariff-tables-july-2012.pdf

    your personal statement: www.ucas.com/how-it-all-works/undergraduate/filling-your-application/your-personal-statement

Unistats: http://unistats.direct.gov.uk.

Chapter 10

Professional regulation

Your licence to practise

Suzan Smallman

In order to work as a nurse in the United Kingdom you must have a 'licence' to practise. This is called 'professional registration' and it is the role of the Nursing and Midwifery Council (NMC) to manage this process. Without registering with the NMC it is illegal to call yourself a 'registered nurse' and practise as such in the UK.

The Nursing and Midwifery Council is a statutory body, established through legislation, whose remit covers all four countries of the United Kingdom. Its primary purpose is to safeguard the health and well-being of the public. This can be confusing to some nurses, as they believe that as they must be registered or licensed to practise with the NMC, it must represent their interests and needs. This however is the role of nursing and midwifery unions (who act on behalf of their members), rather than the role of the NMC, whose main priority is the public and their safety.

The Nursing and Midwifery Council fulfil their role in three ways, by:

1 setting standards for nurses and midwives to get on the register in order that they can practise;
2 setting standards for them to stay on the register;
3 setting standards to remove individuals from the register, as and when necessary.

Through these standards the NMC go some way to ensure that nurses and midwives are safe to practise and remain so throughout their careers.

What is the register?

The register is a list of nurses, midwives and health visitors who are able to practise in the United Kingdom. It is broken into different parts – sub-registers and recordable qualifications.

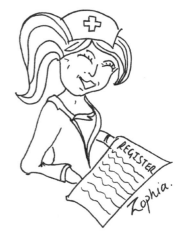

Each registrant's name has a mark alongside it which denotes the field of training undertaken by them, such as child, adult, mental health or learning disability. Some registrants will have trained in several fields and all these are listed alongside their name.

In addition to the register there are some qualifications which can be recorded. These are not required in order for a nurse to practise as a registered nurse but they are ones whereby the nurse must achieve certain NMC standards in order for them to be recognised.

Getting on the register

In the first instance the NMC set standards for education (NMC 2010a) which ensures that all nurses and midwives who wish to practise achieve a level of competence at the point of registration. This is the actual education and training that you have undertaken to be a nurse or a midwife. Each university in the UK has to reach educational standards, set by the NMC, in its pre-registration training programmes (NMC 2010a). These are monitored by the NMC who, through their agents, review the theory and practice delivered by the programme provider and their practice partners. This is to ensure that each programme offered enables students to be competent and be of good health and character when they first register (NMC 2010a). This is sometimes referred to as being 'fit for practice' and 'fit for award'. That is why you will undergo stringent assessment in both practice and theory to ensure that you achieve the standards.

Nurses may apply to register when they first qualify, and they must do this within 5 years of completing an educational programme, otherwise they will lose the right to register without further education. Other nurses who have previously registered but for some reason have had an interruption in practice can re-register, as long as certain criteria are fulfilled. They are required to undertake a Return to Practice course, which is explained in more detail below.

Nurses who trained overseas can apply for UK registration, but they have to demonstrate that the education and training they undertook in their country is equal to that of the UK, and that they have achieved the same standards as those individuals trained in the UK. This doesn't mean that the programmes that overseas nurses have undertaken are of a lesser standard – they may just be different to the requirements of the UK and its healthcare systems.

Staying on the register

In order to for you to remain on the register and thus be deemed safe to practise you need to demonstrate, to the NMC, that you are continuing to work within 'the code' (NMC 2008) and that you are keeping your skills and knowledge up to date.

A recent review of the code has seen some key changes which are set to come into effect on 31 March 2015. This revised code outlines four key themes:

1 prioritise people;
2 practise effectively;
3 preserve safety;
4 and promote professionalism and trust.

It places focus on fundamentals of care, duty of candour, raising concerns, delegation and accountability, professional duty to take action in emergencies and the use of social media (www.nmc-uk.org/Documents/NMC-Publications/NMC-Code-A5-FINAL.pdf).

You are required to register every three years with the NMC and confirm with them that you remain up to date. This is done by:

• Confirming that you have undertaken both 450 hours of registered practice and 35 hours of learning activity in the previous three years (NMC 2011).

- Completing a notification to practice form, confirming that you wish to continue to practise. Again, this is required every three years.
- Paying an annual registration fee.

Post-registration education and practice (Prep)

In order to demonstrate continuing professional development, as nurses you need to enhance your knowledge and skill in both theory and practice throughout your career.

This can be achieved in a number of ways. Examples of theoretical learning activity or academic continuing professional development include:

- attending study days
- undertaking formal postgraduate courses
- participating in online learning
- maintaining a professional portfolio.

There is no set activity and it is the responsibility of each nurse to undertake whatever is applicable to him/her. More detail and examples are provided in *The Prep Handbook*, available from the NMC (2011).

Practice hours do not have to be demonstrated solely through direct patient care, although this is a valid example. Working in research, teaching or management posts are also roles which are equally suitable ways of achieving the required practice hours. Again this often seems confusing to some nurses as they interpret 'practice' as being only direct patient care. This is not the case, as there are many roles which, by virtue of the skills needed, require you to have registration as a nurse.

The NMC is currently reviewing the revalidation process which enables nurses to remain on the register. It is undertaking a full consultation in conjunction with the NMC code (2008; the revised code is due to come into effect from 31 March 2015) which will culminate in some changes to Prep requirements. These changes are set to come into force in December 2015.

Those individuals who cannot demonstrate the practice hours and learning activity and yet want to be registered as a nurse will have to undertake a Return to Practice course. This is a recognised course, usually delivered in a university with support from a Trust, which enables the nurse to renew their skills and demonstrate they are fit to be re-entered on the register.

Good health and character

In completing a notification to practice form as nurses, you are also confirming that you are of good health and character. This demonstrates that you are able to work in a safe and effective manner.

Good health

Good health demonstrates that you are well enough to undertake the duties of a nurse which would not put patients or colleagues at risk. When considering this, you should think about both your physical and mental well-being.

Good character

The role of a nurse requires each of us to work within a code. One of the standards in the code states:

> Be open and honest, act with integrity and uphold the reputation of your profession.
> (NMC 2008: 2)

This clearly identifies that nurses must behave in a way which means that the public will see them as a person who is trustworthy and in whom they have confidence. This requires the nurse to be accountable for their actions, both within employment and in some cases how they portray themselves on a daily basis. For instance they must declare any police charges, cautions or convictions. These are considered as serious matters by the NMC because they reflect upon both the character of the individual and the reputation of the profession. Any nurse reporting a criminal issue has their case referred to a 'Fitness to Practice Committee' to determine whether any action needs to be taken.

Removal from the register

There are a number of circumstances where a nurse is not classed as 'registered' due to having their name removed from the register. Examples are self-removal or removal by the NMC. In both instances the nurse still remains qualified as their academic qualification still stands. It does however mean that the nurse is not licensed to practise as a registered nurse.

Some nurses may choose to remove themselves from the register due to their personal circumstances. For instance they may want to pursue a different career or they may be retiring and thus they will not be able to fulfil the notification to practice requirements. This means that their registration has lapsed, but it does not prevent them from re-registering in the future – it will just mean that they may need to undertake a Return to Practice course in order to fulfil the registration requirements.

There are however circumstances whereby the Nursing and Midwifery Council can remove a nurse from the register. This only happens in serious cases of:

- misconduct
- lack of competence
- character issues
- poor health.

Misconduct

Misconduct is when a nurse's behaviour falls below a standard that could be reasonably expected. For instance, this is in a situation where the nurse has disregarded or not followed the code and thus has compromised the safety of a patient or client.

Lack of competence

A lack of competence is classed as a situation where the nurse or midwife has a lack of knowledge or skill which again affects the safety of the patient or client.

This is usually where the nurse consistently demonstrates a lack of knowledge or skill over a period of time and appears unaware of their lack of competence. An example would be an inability to correctly calculate medication, thus potentially giving incorrect dosages.

Character issues

These are issues whereby it is questioned whether the nurse involved is a good representative of the profession. This often applies where the nurse has been charged and is subsequently given a criminal conviction.

Poor health

Sometimes individuals may have long-term ill-health issues which affect their ability to practise and this may compromise the care that they are delivering to patients and clients. The health issue may be a physical or mental illness.

In all these situations the circumstances of the case are fully investigated. The evidence obtained is then reviewed by an Investigating Committee, who consider all the facts. If it is believed there is a case to answer it is then referred to a Conduct and Competence Committee or, if the health of the registrant is the problem, to a Health Committee.

There are a range of sanctions that can be actioned following the outcome of the committee, with removal from the register being the most serious. Those nurses who are removed from the register cannot practise as a registered nurse and any request to have their registration restored can only be considered after a period of five years. This can have significant consequences for a nurse as it will affect their employability. (See Chapter 15 for more information on employability.)

Other sanctions involve suspending a nurse from the register, which is usually for a fixed period of time, or the nurse having to comply with certain conditions to practise.

The code

The code sets out the standards of conduct, performance and ethics that all nurses and midwives are expected to uphold in order to fulfil their role in maintaining public safety (NMC 2015). It gives the public some assurance that the nurses and midwives who are caring for them are working to a consistent safe standard, and it gives nurses and midwives a foundation on which to base their practice. As described above, the revised code is due to come into effect from 31 March 2015.

The revised code will continue to describe your accountability as a professional nurse, and states the actions required in relation to your dealings with patients, clients and colleagues. Although it is a stand-alone document the code should be read alongside other standards and guidance produced by the NMC. Standards and guidance give more detailed information on areas of practice such as standards for medicines management (NMC 2010b), Prep standards (NMC 2011) or guidance on record keeping (NMC 2009).

Summary

Without registration with the NMC you are unable to practise as a registered nurse. Registration gives assurance to the public that you will care for them in a safe manner. It also requires you to be accountable for your practice.

References

Nursing and Midwifery Council (2008) *The Code: Standards of Conduct, Performance and Ethics for Nurses and Midwives*. London: Nursing and Midwifery Council.

Nursing and Midwifery Council (2009) *Record Keeping: Guidance for Nurses and Midwives*. London: Nursing and Midwifery Council.

Nursing and Midwifery Council (2010a) *Standards for Pre-Registration Nursing Education*. London: Nursing and Midwifery Council.

Nursing and Midwifery Council (2010b) *Standards for Medicines Management*. London: Nursing and Midwifery Council.

Nursing and Midwifery Council (2011) *The Prep Handbook*. London: Nursing and Midwifery Council.

Nursing and Midwifery Council (2015) *The Code: Professional Standards of Practice and Behaviour for Nurses and Midwives*. London: Nursing and Midwifery Council.

Further reading

Siviter, B. (2013) *The Student Nurse Handbook: A Survival Guide*, 3rd Edn. Edinburgh: Bailliere Tindall.

Useful web link

Nursing and Midwifery Council: www.nmc-uk.org.

Chapter 11

Returning to nursing practice

Tim Badger

Most of the chapters in this book are for people who are thinking about joining the nursing profession. But if you have already trained as a nurse and are thinking about returning to nursing after a break – then this chapter is for you. Perhaps you are reading this book because you know someone who is thinking of training, and you have started thinking about nursing again for your own career. Even though you're not practising as a nurse at the moment you may still think of yourself as a nurse, and using some of the caring skills and healthcare knowledge from your nursing experience may still be part of your life.

Keogh (2014) recorded that over 90,000 nurses let their NMC registration lapse in the previous five years, and that as many as 25,725 left the nursing profession within the previous 12 months. If you are one of these ex-registrants and are now considering returning to practice, then read on – as this chapter will point you in the right direction.

The Nursing and Midwifery Council sets standards for what nurses must do to maintain their registration and be able to practise as nurses. Currently this requires periodic re-registration every three years and payment of an annual retention fee. To be eligible for periodic re-registration the nurse must meet the requirements of the NMC (2011) post-registration education and practice (Prep) standards, which specify that in the last three years you must have completed 35 hours of learning activity relevant to your practice, and completed at least 450 hours of registered practice as a nurse. If you do not meet those requirements you cannot re-register, your registration will lapse, and you can no longer practise as a nurse. You may feel that with all your experience you are still a nurse inside, and your friends may look at the way you relate to people and say 'once a nurse, always a nurse', but you will need to complete a Return to Practice programme if you want to practise as a registered nurse again. The NMC, like universities and colleges, uses the word 'programme' to describe what you (and most people) call a 'course'.

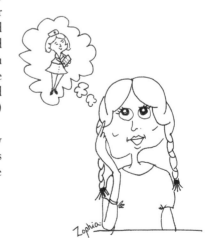

The Nursing and Midwifery Council are currently working on new standards for revalidation. This revalidation process is currently being piloted in the following organisations:

- Aneurin Bevan University Health Board
- Guy's and St Thomas' NHS Foundation Trust

- Mersey Care NHS Trust
- NHS Tayside, and local partners
- Public Health England
- Western Health and Social Care Trust.

It is anticipated that these pilot sites will help identify any ways in which the NMC should refine and define the revalidation model, the guidance required and the associated forms to be used during the revalidation process, prior to its introduction at the end of 2015.

'Revalidation' means that to maintain their registration nurses will need to demonstrate that they are still fit and safe to practise, and that their skills and knowledge are up to date and specific to their current area of practice and role. These requirements will enable the profession to promote a culture of continuous improvement in nursing practice. The NMC is also considering adopting a system (a competency-based test) for nurses wanting to re-join the register similar to the one which came into force for overseas registrants in 2014.

Why did you leave? Why do you want to return?

There are many reasons why nurses choose to leave nursing. Twenty-five years ago the main reason for leaving was the difficulties of combining motherhood with the demands of working as a nurse, a pattern which reflected the predominance of young women in the profession. Nowadays, family commitments are still one of the main reasons why people stop working as nurses, but changes in society and increased opportunities for family-friendly working mean that these commitments are not just childcare. It may be that the need to support ageing parents or care for a sick partner or sibling was the family commitment that led you to lapse your nursing registration.

'Freedom to return' is a common reason people give for returning to nursing, but if you left nursing due to family commitments you need to be sure that now is the right time for you to return, and that you will be able to meet the commitments of working as a nurse again as well as your personal commitments. It is important to find out what the demands of nursing are now, such as the shift patterns in hospital. One of the effects of government policies to provide 'care in the community' and 'move care closer to home' has been an expansion in community services that are provided around the clock.

A second reason why people leave nursing is a change in career. The boundaries between health and social care have shifted over the years and it may be that your career has led you into roles which no longer required you to be registered as a nurse, either as a practitioner or as a manager, and that now you think your next career step will be one that requires you to be registered again as a nurse. Some people leave nursing to train for a related career, such as midwifery (although many midwives do maintain their nurse registration as well), or to train in a career such as teaching or social work, where the people skills they developed in nursing would be invaluable. Redundancy or reorganisation in their new career is a common reason that people think about nursing again.

It may be that you left nursing for other family reasons – quite a few returners say they left nursing to work in a family business. Other family reasons for leaving are to do with family relocation – perhaps you've lived abroad in a country where you'd not learnt enough of the language to feel you could nurse, or moved to a remote part of the UK where opportunities to use hospital nursing experience are limited.

Some returning nurses give 'salary' as their reason for returning to nursing – perhaps the alternative career path you have followed has not paid as well as you had hoped. Perhaps you hope that renewing your registration as a nurse will take you into another area of work, such as health visiting. Or perhaps you have a feeling of 'unfinished business', in that you remember that nursing had given you a feeling of personal satisfaction and self-worth that another career has not met, and you now feel that the experiences you have had will give you extra skills to offer in nursing.

Or maybe you left nursing because there was something about it that you did not like. 'Shift work', 'feeling underpaid and undervalued', 'stressed by the clinical environment', 'ill health', 'short-staffing', and 'feeling unsupported at work' are all reasons nurses give for leaving the profession. If you are thinking about returning to nursing it is important to be honest with yourself about why you left. If you left for negative reasons, you need to think about whether things are really going to be different this time.

What is a Return to Practice programme?

The NMC Prep (NMC 2011) standards require Return to Practice programmes to be offered by universities which the NMC have approved to provide them. The Prep standards set nine outcomes that the programme must provide:

1 an understanding of the influence of health and social policy relevant to the practice of nursing and midwifery;
2 an understanding of the requirements of legislation, guidelines, codes of practice and policies relevant to the practice of nursing and midwifery;
3 an understanding of the current structure and organisation of care, nationally and locally;
4 an understanding of current issues in nursing and midwifery education and practice;
5 the use of relevant literature and research to inform the practice of nursing and midwifery;
6 the ability to identify and assess need, design and implement interventions and evaluate outcomes in all relevant areas of practice, including the effective delivery of appropriate emergency care;
7 the ability to use appropriate communications, teaching and learning skills;
8 the ability to function effectively in a team and participate in a multi-professional approach to people's care;
9 the ability to identify strengths and weaknesses, acknowledge limitations of competence, and recognise the importance of maintaining and developing professional competence.

(NMC 2011: 7)

The Prep standards state that a Return to Practice programme will be not less than five days in length, but when you look at the outcomes you can see that although some can be achieved through university study, there are others which can only be achieved by time in practice. The NMC do not specify how long you need to spend in practice on a Return to Practice programme, and that varies between programmes. Most specify a minimum number of hours – many say 150 hours, which would be four weeks full-time, or ten weeks if you do two 7.5-hour shifts per week.

Return to Practice programmes require you to pass an assessment, usually covering both theory and practice. The theory assessment might be an assignment or developing a portfolio, and the practice assessment might be providing evidence that you have met the required outcomes, that you know what you are doing and why you are doing it, and that you can do it. The NMC require that to re-join the register you need to be assessed by a 'sign-off mentor' – a nurse from the same field of nursing as yourself who has completed the additional training and experience to assess practice proficiency at the end of an NMC-approved programme. The main role for a sign-off mentor is assessing student nurses at the end of their training as competent or proficient to practise safely and effectively without supervision, and the sign-off mentor will need to make the same judgement of competence about you. This requirement to be assessed by a sign-off mentor means that you will need to have the flexibility to be able to commit to working regularly with your sign-off mentor during the course. For you, being signed-off by a mentor should give you confidence that in becoming a registered nurse you have shown yourself to be fit to practise.

A Return to Practice programme can only return you to the same part of the register as you were on previously. So if you originally trained as an adult or general nurse you must gain your practice experience and be assessed by a sign-off mentor in an adult nursing environment. Even if you've worked in some capacity in mental health services whilst your nursing registration has lapsed, you can only return to adult nursing. Further information relating to NMC registration can be found in Chapter 10.

How do I find a Return to Practice programme?

Return to Practice programmes must be approved by the Nursing and Midwifery Council, so the first place to start is their website (www.nmc-uk.org) which provides details of the universities they have approved. The section of the website on registration includes information on 'Returning to Practice' and there is a link from there to the list of universities who provide the courses. Don't just look for the university nearest to you as some offer their courses at campuses in more than one town. They may also offer part of the course by distance learning, which might suit you if you live in a remote rural part of the country, and you should be able to do the practice experience closer to home.

The NMC list can seem quite confusing. As well as the names of the universities it has other information, such as 'level 3' or 'level 5'. This refers to the academic level of the course, not to the professional level of your nursing qualification, which describes Enrolled Nurse qualifications as level 2. The levels are confusing as different universities use different systems to describe the academic level of their courses. Where a course is described as level 2 or level 5 in England and Wales, or level 8 in Scotland, it will be delivered at diploma level, and if it is described as level 3, level 6 or level 9 it will be delivered at degree level.

The next stage is to find out about the programme offered by each university. Each university will have its own website where you will find some general information about their course – using the phrases 'return to practice' or 'return to nursing' in the website's search box will find you information, or you may be able to download a prospectus or contact a course enquiries team. After seeing the information on the website you will almost certainly want to get information from someone who is involved with running the course, either a tutor or course administrator. You can contact them by phone or email, or by going to an open day advertised on the website.

The other way you might find out information is from your local hospitals or community healthcare organisations. Within NHS Trusts there will usually be a Professional Development team, or staff with titles like 'Practice Educator' or 'Practice Education Facilitator/Manager'. These people can advise you about how their organisation can support you in returning to practice and about their links with the universities who provide programmes (but they will also suggest you contact a university about the course yourself).

What do I need to find out about the Return to Practice programme?

Before you phone someone up, send them an email or go to an open day. It is a good idea to have thought beforehand about what you want to know. Below are some common questions you might like to find out the answers to, so that you can make an informed decision about whether a Return to Practice programme is right for you at the present time.

How long is a Return to Practice programme?

This will depend on your shift pattern on placement and how quickly you pass all the assessments. It might be possible to complete the course in a couple of months, but most returners will typically take three to six months.

Will I need to pay for the programme myself?

This varies between different parts of the UK. Funding is currently (2014) available for returning to nursing in Wales but not in England. There is no fixed price for a Return to Practice programme and fees vary between universities. Unless you are being sponsored to return to practice you will need to complete the practice placement hours in your own time and you will not be paid for attending the placement.

Why do some programmes say I need to find my own placement?

In areas where Return to Practice programmes are not paid for by the NHS, placements are not part of an existing contract between the NHS and the university. Although the programme tutor requires you to do some work in finding your own placement he or she should still be able to help you with suggestions of people to approach. Asking about placements gives an opportunity to discuss personal needs (part time or full time, shift patterns) and also helps you find out about future employment prospects.

Can I do the placement in a nursing home or with my local GP's practice nurse?

The university will need to confirm that the suggested placement can meet NMC standards in providing a suitable learning environment, supervision and a sign-off mentor, and provide you with the necessary experience to meet the Return to Practice outcomes. If a practice area provides nursing students with their final placement of their training it should be able to meet these requirements – a nursing home may be able to do this, a practice nurse probably not.

I've lapsed my registration as both a nurse and a health visitor. Do I need to do a return to nursing programme to go back to health visiting?

To be registered as a Health Visitor (or other Specialist Community Public Health Nurse) you also need to be registered as a nurse or midwife. The NMC no longer approve separate 'Return to Health Visiting' programmes, so you need to do a return to nursing or midwifery programme which includes a heath visiting component to meet your needs. The government committed to substantially increase the number of health visitors by 2015, and in 2011 funding was made available for health visiting returners.

I was an Enrolled Nurse – do I need to do a different Return to Practice programme?

Return to Practice programmes are the same for second-level (enrolled) and first-level nurses. As an Enrolled Nurse it is a good idea to find out about your employment opportunities after re-registration. 'Conversion courses' no longer exist, so if your longer-term aim is to become a first-level nurse you would need to do part of a three-year programme. In this case, ask the university about its accreditation procedures to decide what is the best route for you.

I've not studied for years, and when I trained it was at a hospital school of nursing. Will I cope at a university?

Some programmes will want you to have done recent study as an entry requirement or advise specific preparation before starting. Most universities offer study skills support for things like essay writing, information literacy, and preparing for job applications and interviews as part of the programme, and also as part of their service to all students who want extra support. If the Return to Practice programme offers a choice of diploma or degree level module, consider which one is more suitable for you. Unless you have already got a diploma or degree, a diploma-level module will be more suitable for you.

I've lost all my old certificates. How can I show I used to be a nurse?

The Nursing and Midwifery Council's Registrations Department can provide you with a statement of entry which shows that your registration has lapsed.

Will I need to provide references?

Getting a place on a programme will require references to be taken up as well as Occupational Health and Disclosure and Barring Service (DBS) checks. The programme tutor will recognise that if you have not been employed for six years, you cannot provide a meaningful employer's reference, and may discuss with you who you could approach instead. At the end of the programme you will need to provide two good character references to the Nursing and Midwifery Council in addition to the programme tutor, so if you cannot provide references to get on the programme you would have trouble re-registering at the end.

Are there any 'hidden costs' as well as the programme fee?

A Return to Practice programme will require DBS and Occupational Health checks, and wearing a uniform, so you should find out whether these are included in the programme fee or are additional costs. Universities generally have good libraries, with many resources available online as e-books and e-journals, as well as online learning sites, so you will want to have regular internet access. You should find out about costs associated with your placement – hospital car parking is usually not free.

Summary

If you are seriously considering becoming a registered nurse again I hope this chapter has given you a good insight into what you need to do. If you left due to the stresses of being a nurse, please be mindful that those stressors are more than likely still evident, along with potentially new stressors. So it is really important that you embark on your return to nursing programme with your eyes wide open – without looking back with rose-tinted spectacles. Be clear about your reasons for wanting to return to the nursing profession and, importantly, be prepared for theory and practice challenges as you take that step back on to the professional register.

References

Keogh, K. (2014) The NHS needs you – call goes out to nurses who left the profession. *Nursing Standard* 28(39): 14–15.
Nursing and Midwifery Council (2011) *The Prep Handbook*. London: Nursing and Midwifery Council.

Further reading

Nursing and Midwifery Council (2008) *Standards to Support Learning and Assessment in Practice*. London: Nursing and Midwifery Council.

Useful web link

Nursing and Midwifery Council: www.nmc-uk.org.

Part 4

What and where you will learn

Chapter 12

Life in university

Carol Doyle, Bethann Siviter and Cathy Poole

Nursing programmes funded by the National Health Service (NHS) differ from other university degrees, as not only are they governed by university rules and regulations but also by the Nursing and Midwifery Council (NMC) which is the professional regulatory and statutory body.

The course can run over three years or four years. It is important to consider which course is best for you – the real difference is that the longer course follows a more traditional academic year.

Half of your programme will be in the university, whilst the other half will be spent in clinical placements – within NHS, private and voluntary healthcare settings in the community, hospital or other healthcare delivery areas relevant to your own and other branches – to ensure that you develop well-rounded practical abilities supported by your academic development. At the start of the course, you have more academic time than placement time, so you have time to build a solid foundation in theoretical nursing. As the course progresses, you will shift to more placement time, so that at the end of the course, you rarely go to university. This will help you make that eventual transition from student to qualified nurse.

You will attend classes (there will be a set number of modules in each university period) but also have self-directed learning, so that you can build on your experiences in placement and with other students to expand your learning. As a nurse, reflection and self-development are essential, so both are important from the very start of your nursing career – you must be disciplined enough to learn from your experiences without a tutor looking over your shoulder, and you must take the time you need to prepare for papers, for clinical placements and for exams. So do not fritter your self-directed learning time on other things!

The modules in your programme will give you the basics of nursing and the elements essential for safe, effective and professional nursing care. You will work with students from your own and other fields from the start to ensure that you develop awareness beyond just your own field of study. Patients don't just have health problems in one area – and just as their needs extend outside the boundaries of our nursing branches, so must your awareness.

Your clinical experience is similar to how your life will be when you work. You will work 37.5 hours a week in practice, and are expected to follow the same type of shift patterns as nurses do – long days, nights, weekends and late shifts, followed by 'earlies'. You will need to manage your travel to ensure you are on time. If, due to caring commitments or disability, you can't work certain shifts or shift patterns, it is essential you speak in advance to both your university and to your mentor, as the NMC guidance guarantees you reasonable adjustments. Despite this, you must show that you develop proficiency in care around the clock so, if there is an issue, work with your university to ensure that you fully develop the skills and knowledge you require. This is explained in further detail below.

If there are problems with travel, consider asking around. There will be other staff and other students who are also travelling, and they may be willing to share a lift with you.

In summary, the nursing programme is different from other university programmes due to its clinical placements and the nature of your development. You are doing more than following an academic course of study – you are developing as a caring, knowledgeable and practically skilled professional nurse.

Academic levels of study

The majority of pre-registration nursing programmes are now what we call graduate programmes. This means that when you qualify you attain a nursing degree. Some programmes are also delivered as Master's courses (level 7) so it is important that you understand which course you are undertaking. Often the Master's programmes are for students who have already got a degree and they apply to undertake an accelerated nursing course over two years. Examples of this can be found on the following web links:

Mental health nursing: www.essex.ac.uk/coursefinder/course_details.aspx?course—SC+ B74024
Adult nursing: www.brookes.ac.uk/studying-at-brookes/courses/postgraduate/2014/adult-nursing-preregistration
Children's nursing: www.nottingham.ac.uk/ugstudy/courses/nursing/graduate-entry-nursing-child.aspx.

When most students commence their nurse training they will have studied at level 3 (A level equivalent) so now it is time to continue up the academic ladder of learning. What this means is that your assessments during your first year at university will be at the next academic level – level 4. Subsequent years will see you developing your level 5 (diploma) and level 6 (degree) study skills. All universities use a variety of assessment strategies – for example, essays, examinations, objective structured clinical examination (OSCE), presentations, dissertations, etc. This approach makes sure that all students have the opportunity to excel in their assessments.

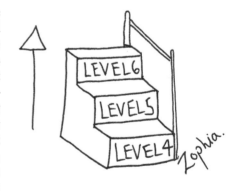

Nursing domains

The NMC (2010) is responsible for setting the standards for pre-registration nurse training. They are currently divided into four 'domains' which are relevant to all fields of nursing:

1   Professional values
2   Communication and interpersonal skills
3   Nursing practice and decision making
4   Leadership, management and team working.

Domain 1: Professional values

Adherence to professional values is a key part of what makes nursing a profession. We have a code of conduct, and there is an expectation that we will follow ethical principles when working with others. We set ourselves a high standard, and promise to achieve it. We don't see people for what makes them different, or treat them according to our values for people of their class, social group or economic standing. We treat all people the same, irrespective of anything other than their health and individual needs. We see people as equal, and deserving of our care (even when others might not).

We act honestly, do not lie, do not hide information, and do not act for our own benefit. We act transparently, and we own up to mistakes when we make them. We speak up when things go wrong, and challenge those whose 'care' hurts our patients. We advocate for our patients, based on our values, but also on up-to-date and evidence-based knowledge and skill. We reflect on our practice in order to improve, and we ensure that we are always ready to do what our patients need.

We must act honestly and respectfully, ensure that those we care for are treated with dignity, and that we tell the truth and follow the law, and that we put the needs of those we care for before anything else.

The Chief Nursing Officer of England set out the '6Cs' as a pattern for nurses but also for healthcare organisations. Although not strictly nursing values, they do set out the way nurses should behave, and the priorities nurses should have. The 6Cs are:

1   Care: we will help individuals and communities to experience the care they need. People have a right to receive consistent care throughout their lives, and to be treated in a manner than feels 'caring' to them.
2   Compassion: compassion is delivered through empathy, respect and dignity. It is kindness, respect for individual needs and experiences, and shows concern for how the person perceives their care.
3   Competence: the ability of those providing care to understand and meet a person's needs effectively and with awareness of evidence and best practice.
4   Communication: listening and helping others to understand their experiences. Working effectively with others, expressing oneself verbally, non-verbally and in writing. Effective and sensitive communication underpins effective care.
5   Courage: speaking up and escalating concerns, whistleblowing and challenging others are all part of courage in care. It requires both vision and strength, as well as being willing to change, to demonstrate courage in caring.
6   Commitment: a genuine commitment to patients starts with the desire to improve their well-being, give a good experience, and focus on their needs as they perceive them.

The code for nurses and midwives, which has recently been revised and is due to come into effect on 31 March 2015 (NMC 2015), and the guidance for students (NMC 2011) are both outlined on the NMC website. Be familiar with them, as they are the yardstick against which your practice will be measured – from your first days as a student to your last days as a nurse.

In summary, as a nurse, you must provide care to people, irrespective of their background, their religion, colour, disability, sexual orientation or anything else that makes them different. You must always be worthy of trust, and do the right thing, even when it is difficult or when others don't agree. Your core values, as well as those of the organisation for which you work, must comply with the values expected through the NMC and the regulatory guidance for healthcare and, together, these values drive the way you work, communicate and care. The values you show in daily practice are the cornerstone of professional practice – without them, you cannot be a nurse.

Domain 2: Communication and interpersonal skills

Communication is the single most substantial skill you need to develop to work effectively as a nurse. Here are some typical areas where good communication is essential:

- Gaining consent for a procedure or for care
- Assessing a patient's condition and needs
- Documenting care and treatment
- Talking to carers and families
- Sharing concerns with colleagues
- Delegating tasks or receiving delegation
- Getting help to complete a task.

Everything you do involves communication. But you cannot always control what other people perceive about your thoughts and feelings. Your body language might say something other than your words, and if it does, another person is more likely to believe what your body language says rather than your words. So you need to be aware of – and control – your non-verbal communication.

You need to learn the basics of clinical communication, but you also need to hone your customer-service skills to ensure that you behave appropriately. Ask yourself, 'How would I feel and what would I want from a nurse if this were me? Or my Mum or Dad?' Watch the way professionals communicate, and if you find their style particularly effective, reassuring or caring, speak to them and ask how they developed their style. Find someone who makes you feel badly. Look at what they do and how, and reflect on how easy it is to behave the same way. As a student, use every experience to further your learning. Even a bad experience can provide a good outcome.

Reflecting on your actions – both good and bad – will help you learn. What are some of the most problematic elements of communication that you must avoid? Box 12.1 might help you.

Passive aggressiveness is a big problem as it often results from stress. It is when you say something that sounds OK at face value, but everyone knows it is not what is meant. Saying 'I'd work with you anytime' whilst rolling your eyes makes it clear that you mean the opposite of what you are saying. Passive aggressiveness is the absolute depth of unprofessional and ineffective communication, and you should avoid it.

One really important thing in professional communication can be forgotten – even by those with experience: listen to and believe your patient. See each person with fresh eyes,

---

Box 12.1 Elements of communication to be avoided

- Not making eye contact
- Eye-rolling
- Deep sighing
- Failing to remember that people can hear you even when asleep, or with an altered level of consciousness (anaesthesia, coma, etc.)
- Not listening to what people say, or only hearing what you want to hear
- Intentionally avoiding speaking with people
- Using your hands to motion 'hurry up'
- Passive aggressiveness
- Smirking
- Teeth-sucking
- Speaking to someone other than the patient when the patient is in your company
- Judging people or making assumptions about them based on name, appearance, diagnosis, or some other subjective issue
- Calling people 'dear', 'duckie', 'sweetie', instead of using their name
- Saying dismissive things like 'yes, yes' to hush someone
- Using the term 'whatever' when people express concerns.

---

and use your knowledge and skill to determine their needs. Pay attention to them, and don't assume you or anyone else knows more about their needs than they do. If your patient says 'I'm in pain', then they are in pain, no matter what anyone else says. Document what the patient says, what you see, and then do what needs to be done.

Respect that others may know more about the patient than you or your team does. If the patient's family member says 'Something's wrong' then, also, listen and find out. There are countless cases of a complaint following a terrible situation, where the family member says 'I told you – why didn't you listen to me?' Don't be the one who didn't listen. Your communication skills, networks and knowledge must be used to advocate for your patients and to meet their needs.

Ask colleagues about your communication style, and when you reflect, ask them to give feedback on your style. Do they always feel you listen? Do they feel you show caring?

In summary, remember that communication is a tool. You must not take its value for granted, and take care to ensure you only communicate what you intend to communicate, whether in writing, in speech or non-verbally. Skilled professionals have professional communication skills. It is the one skill you absolutely must develop to be successful.

Domain 3: Nursing practice and decision making

Nursing practice is based on nursing theory – nurses use theories and evidence to make decisions. The 'nursing process' (assessment, planning, implementation and evaluation) is a way of thinking and approaching care that aids decision making. It does not tell you what to do – it tells you how to decide what to do. You will learn about the theories and models that nurses use, and these will help you with your assessment and decision making. The nursing process is a good tool, and can be used from the very start of your course. Remember APIE: Assessment, Planning, Implementation and Evaluation.

Assessment

What is the situation? What are the person's needs? What does the person want and what does the person say? What do I see and what can I measure or objectively determine? Who else should be involved? What are the clinical issues, medications, diagnoses, etc.? Your answers will lead to: 'These are the problems I must resolve.'

Planning

What do I need to achieve? What is possible? What is not possible? How can I bring the current situation to a more desirable situation? How can I avoid the common pitfalls or problems that commonly occur in situations like this? Who else needs to be involved?

Implementation

What are the specific actions and steps needed to bring this problem to a conclusion, in the most positive way possible? Who else needs to be involved? When do I (or someone else) need to step in to re-assess the situation?

Evaluation

How will I determine if the implementation has successfully resolved the problems? Using 'SMART goals' (Box 12.2) I must state the outcomes which I desire and how they can be assessed.

Decision making

Other professionals diagnose – they look at the patient's physical condition and decide what's wrong. Nurses don't diagnose. They assess. They look at the patient's needs and abilities, and decide the help and support they need to be as independent as possible.

To make good decisions, you should use your communication skills to gather information to ensure that you have a good understanding of the problem and the possible resolution. If you lack experience, seek guidance from someone who knows more, and then make a plan to improve your knowledge.

When finding a way forward, it helps to start at the end result. Think about the most desirable situation for the person and the circumstances in which you are involved – and then plan backwards to determine how to get there.

In summary, your decision making is informed by:

- The patient and their perspective
- Resources you can access (including your team and specialists)
- Understanding of the patient's problems, needs and circumstances and planning what can be done to meet their needs effectively.

Box 12.2 SMART goals

SMART goals are useful in a wide range of areas, and commonly used in business and science. You will use SMART goals repeatedly during your education and eventual career! SMART goals are:

Specific: A simple, concise statement that outlines what the resolved problem looks like.

Measurable: The success of the outcome can be clearly measured.

Achievable: The outcome has to be something that can be achieved – and there should be a specific person who is named for each action to ensure that it gets done.

Reasonable: Not only is it achievable, it is a reasonable thing to expect.

Timed (or timely): There are two parts. How long will this goal take to achieve? and Will it be achieved in steps (sub-goals) or in one jump?

Example
The issue is: A patient has slippers that don't fit and, as a result, it is hard for them to walk safely.

S: The patient will have slippers that fit well to ensure safe walking.

M: Current slippers are size L. European size 36 slippers would be appropriate and not slip off the feet when the patient walks.

A: The patient's daughter will purchase the slippers.

R: Appropriate slippers are needed for safe walking. If slippers cannot be purchased, trainers will be needed.

T: This goal must be achieved within 24 hours.

Domain 4: Leadership, management and team working

Leaders and managers have similar responsibilities but different approaches. They are linked by the need to ensure the best direction for an organisation and its staff. It is not easy to separate them: every leader needs management understanding, and every manager needs leadership. They both need to understand basic principles of 'workplace hygiene' – the way people work, what drives them to do well, and what causes problems. You don't need to be an expert to be a leader; understanding leadership will help you build leadership skills throughout your course and career.

In his book, *On Becoming a Leader*, Bennis (2009) wrote a sensible list that outlines the differences between managers and leaders (see Box 12.3).

When thinking about management, you need to think about more than getting the job done. Managers need to have a sense of the big picture – from the economic issues to the

BOX 12.3 Differences between managers and leaders (after Bennis 2009)

Managers	Leaders
Administers	Innovates
Is as other managers	Is original
Maintains the status quo	Develops new ideas
Focuses on systems and structures	Focuses on people
Relies on control	Inspires trust
Short range view	Long range perspective
Asks: How and When	Asks: What and Why
Sees the bottom line	Sees the horizon
Imitates other managers	Originates their style
Accepts the status quo	Challenges the status quo
Is a good soldier	Is his or her own person
In summary, the manager does things right.	In summary, the leader does the right thing.

personnel matters that impact staff. Leaders also have a sense of a big picture, but it is more about what could happen than what does presently. They must see the world that could exist, and inspire people to buy in and follow them. Whilst leaders inspire and innovate, managers organise and assign. Together, managers and leaders help people do the right things to ensure the workplace is effective.

How can you be a leader, even as a student? Do the right things, support other people, and concern yourself with learning to be an effective, caring and skilled nurse. If you read back on the list of what makes a leader, you will see that every single attribute comes from a sense of hope for a better future, and the desire to improve things for those in our care.

Although every professional should aspire to be a leader, good management skills get the work done. Being able to organise your work, prioritise your activity and manage your time are all essential skills that add to your clinical abilities. As you advance in your career, you will learn additional management skills, like being able to develop an effective 'off-duty' (schedule) for your staff, to appraise staff performance and prepare budget and other business reports. But without leadership, you will not have the credibility you need to be seen as an effective manager and nurse.

In summary, both leadership and management are important, but together they give you a good skill set to provide, lead and organise good care. Leaders and managers are both made, not born – you must learn both skill sets as part of your nursing development.

Academic support and study skills

Academic support will come from three areas – and there is a fourth source of academic support that you must avoid.

First, you will get support from your tutors and your personal tutor. You will get guidance in the form of a 'Module Guide' or outline, listing the learning outcomes, the expected teaching pathways, a timeline, how the module will be assessed, and the suggested resources you should use. You can meet with your tutor to discuss the assessment of the module, and get feedback on your progress. You should make appointments in advance to ensure that your tutor's time is available for you. Come prepared for tutorials – many tutors will not have read full papers, but will have read outlines and plans. Hint – if tutors list three books on their Module Guide, they want you to use them in the assignment for their module!

Second, the university will have resources in addition to tutors. Libraries, National Student Union, and peer study groups are all common academic support routes. The library is always going to be the best place to start. There are often guides on a wide range of topics, including referencing, study skills and everything else you need to be successful.

Third, your peers on the course are a valuable resource. Discuss issues with them, learn from and with them – but don't copy from them or do work in common with them when individual work is required. This leads to the thing you must avoid: plagiarism.

Plagiarism is copying work, buying work off the internet, trying to pass papers off as your own when they really came from someone else. All of these things will cause you to lose your place on the course, and once labelled a cheater you won't get into another course. (Don't think you won't get caught, because you will – there are software packages that scan papers to make sure they are original.) You need to stand before your patient as a nurse. If you have not done the work, you do not earn the title. But that does not mean friends cannot help you learn – it just means you must learn on your own!

There are some things that will make your academic development much easier:

1   Plan ahead and build study time into your schedule. Write papers over a longer period, setting landmarks in your diary. Waiting until the last minute deprives you of the support and help you might have had otherwise.
2   Show up, pay attention in class, and don't disturb others. Turn your phone off and be attentive. Even the most boring lecture will help you, although it might take work. Chatting, texting, surfing and fooling around hurt your own and others' development. If you want to be respected as a professional, act like one from the first day of the course.
3   Take notes and organise your class notes and resources to ensure that you can review them and use them to prepare for assessment. If you don't know how to take notes, learn – the library can help you.
4   Know the learning outcomes you are expected to achieve. If you write a brilliant paper that does not show the learning outcomes, the paper will fail. If you are not sure if the paper will show what you need it to, ask your tutor.
5   Spell-check your work and use the correct format, grammar and terminology when you write. You will lose points for poor spelling. How would you feel about the credibility of this book if you read 'Mek sure u has good study skillz sose youse can be a Nuse'?
6   Don't fib or make stuff up. Your tutor knows the resources they have recommended, and if they see something that seems unusual, they will check it.
7   Use the correct referencing format and reference all your sources – this shows respect for those who have aided your development through sharing their knowledge. Failure in this area is so avoidable – many libraries have electronic templates to help you format your references properly.

In summary, you can develop study skills before or during your course. The key skills are time management, organisation and planning. You will need resources to help you understand what your tutors want, and organising your information, and meeting with your tutors, will help you spend your time effectively.

Your life as a student (Who are you?)

The information you need to be successful as a nursing student really depends on who you are. There are three groups of people who apply for nursing programmes:

- People who are just finishing their basic education, at age 18–20;
- People who are older, perhaps have worked or raised a family and are now looking to fulfil their dream of becoming a nurse;
- People who have followed other careers but who have now decided to follow nursing.

The experiences, needs and expectations of all of these people will be different. No matter the age or reason you have come to nursing, you will find enrichment and support through your time in university – and you will be supporting others too.

What do you need to think about and what experience might you need to have? You will be dealing with people in what is a very difficult and stressful time in their lives when they are unwell, in pain, feeling vulnerable and perhaps very afraid. They may behave differently than they would if well, and may evoke some very strong feelings in those caring for them. It can be very upsetting to care for people who are ill, suffering, facing major disruptions to their lives or even facing its end. This is called the 'emotional labour' of nursing, and the only real way to know if you can manage it is to have some experience caring for people. Spending some time as a Health Care Support Worker/Health Care Assistant is beneficial for several reasons – it will give you basic skills, an understanding of and respect for what these key staff do, and it will give you an insight into the nature of nursing care and the circumstances in which nurses work.

Those who are older and who have had careers and families may find it difficult to step back to 'beginner' level, but it helps your relationships and development if you can let go of all the responsibilities and control you have experienced in the past and simply allow yourself to develop as a nurse. Your life experiences are invaluable, and will help you and your colleagues to develop into caring, compassionate and skilled nurses.

Those who are entering right from college or at a young age can ask for work experience, or get a job as a carer or Health Care Assistant. This can be achieved through the NHS jobs hub (www.jobs.nhs.uk) or through your local paper (if you want a job outside an NHS entity). But be aware: working in a nursing or care home is valuable and important work, but sometimes the level of care provided may not be the same level expected in an acute hospital. Be careful to reflect on your practice and develop the best possible skills.

One important financial note: as a student nurse, you can get discounts and benefits reserved for students, in areas from banking to insurance to council tax. Make certain to maximise these benefits, and be sure to find out about the National Union of Students and the benefits membership offers! Every penny counts, especially for student nurses.

Joining a union

Most nurses – in fact, most healthcare professionals – belong to a union. There are two main unions for nurses that will actively recruit you as a student: Unison and the Royal College of Nursing. They will each offer you a discount on your membership and a range of benefits. Amongst these benefits are access to student-oriented materials and resources, and representation should you have a problem on placement. Most will also offer you a discount on your eventual membership as a professional.

During your first month at university, these unions will have presentations and displays, offer you freebies and explain how they are the only union to meet your needs. In reality, they are all much the same – a fair few students join both, and then let their experiences guide which one they join when they qualify. Don't see a free dictionary as evidence of a good union – look for concrete support, and match the union with the level of support you think you will need. If you are working as a Health Care Assistant, will your student membership cover you? Is there a discount on a journal? Or access to full text online nursing libraries?

Joining a union is a good idea for students, and the usual membership is only about £10 a year. Get the freebies, then after a year only renew the membership that you see as most beneficial.

Accommodation and travel

As a student nurse, you will live at home or in student digs, at or near the university. Most universities only offer university accommodation to first year students, but there is often a thriving market in student accommodation around universities! If you have never rented accommodation before, bring someone who has with you. There are pitfalls to consider, like parking, access, responsibility for damages, etc. The university often has a housing office that can help you find suitable digs, either alone or shared. Each has its benefits and its issues.

The university can tell you which sites it most commonly uses for placements, and this could impact your choice of housing. Take some time to explore public transport (especially if you do not have a car). You may need to work very early or very late, so note the service's start and stop times. The good news is that as soon as you are a student you can get a student bus pass and railcard, both of which will save you money. The bad news is that parking is always a problem, for staff and students alike. Whether living at home or at university, travel and parking are important considerations, because you must be on time, at university and on placement. Some universities allow only limited parking for students, and some placement areas either have no parking for students, or expect students to pay for parking (just as staff do). You can find out about parking costs in advance, either through a particular trust's website or through direct contact, but expect them to be high. Although driving clearly has its benefits, there are issues as well, so take time to think about the pros and cons before deciding.

Remember that you will have placements in more than one hospital, and that you will work Sundays and Bank Holidays, school holidays and around the clock at times when public transport is limited. Think about your entire programme when planning where to attend and where to live.

Some students have opted for short-term housing near a placement area when travel is too difficult. You can find out about housing of this nature through estate agents who specialise in student and healthcare professional housing needs. It is not cheap, but reduced travel costs and peace of mind can offset the costs.

Disability

If you have special housing, transport, travel or other specific needs due to disability, make sure to discuss them with the university before making any arrangements or decisions. Both the law (the Equality Act in England, Wales and Scotland, and the Disability Discrimination Act in Northern Ireland) and Kane and Gooding's (2009) guidance on behalf of the NMC set out that disabled students should be given 'reasonable adjustments' to ensure they can participate as fully as other students. However you can only exercise your rights if you communicate in advance with the university and make your needs and abilities clear. They cannot help you manage problems that they don't know about.

Just in case you wonder about a disabled student being a nurse, students with a range of problems, including impaired mobility, missing an arm, impaired vision, impaired hearing, depression, with dyslexia and a range of other physical and emotional health issues have successfully become nurses. Disability does not need to be an obstacle. Both law and guidance do give you the right to help if you need it, but only if you let people know what you need.

When will I work? Shift patterns

Universities have an 'allocations' (placement) office that finds and assigns students to clinical placements. Although they are willing to do what they can to help students, they have too many students and too many placements to give each student their exact choice of placement area.

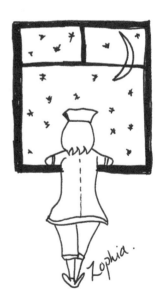

Allocations are provided on a schedule that can vary by university. How to find out where you are allocated is one of the first things you will learn at university. The type of placement will vary to ensure that you have a wide range of the experiences needed for qualification. On each placement, a nurse who has taken a course in supporting students' learning in placements (NMC 2008) will be assigned as a mentor, to both assist you in learning and assess your performance. You should work with your mentor on at least two shifts out of five. In some areas, an additional mentor may also be designated to ensure that you have adequate support and supervision. The 'off-duty' (schedule) is usually available in advance so check it to ensure that you work adequate shifts with your mentor. This is explained in more detail in Chapter 13.

Childcare

Whilst in university, you will have a set timetable for each module for the duration of the module, so you will know what days and times you will attend. This makes planning childcare (or care of a disabled person) much easier to manage and organise. If you do not have childcare arranged, check the university website or ask Student Services if your university has a crèche. The age range of children accepted could vary (as will the costs) and places will be limited. One word of warning – this childcare may become unsuitable when you are on placement as its opening times and distance from placement may make it inappropriate for continued use. It should also be noted that university crèches may be closed or only offer reduced service during university breaks and vacations.

If the university nursery is too expensive or not flexible enough, then you may want to make childcare arrangements nearer to home. This means you may be able to secure a place in an establishment (or with a childminder) that has extended opening hours and is available 52 weeks of the year. Local councils hold registers of childminders and children's nurseries, and quality reports are available on the Ofsted website. Sometimes, student nurses group together and care for each other's children during placements. This only works if the group is large enough to accommodate the various shift demands, but other students can be useful contacts to help in a pinch.

Consult your partner and extended family with regards to working shifts and the implications for childcare, because during weekends, night duty and public holidays you may not be able to find suitable paid-for childcare to meet your needs. Let them know from the start what expectations there are for you, and it will be easier to enjoy their support.

Students may be entitled to financial help with childcare costs from the NHS Bursary Childcare Allowance. Chapter 14 provides more information on financial support. The NHS Bursary Unit (2010) provides further information regarding childcare in their guidance booklet *Help with Childcare Costs for NHS Students*.

If you have caring responsibilities for a disabled person, the law and the NMC guidance both provide that you be given suitable reasonable adjustments. Speak to your university and when on placement with your mentor. If you have any difficulties achieving reasonable adjustments, your university should support you, but remember you must show that you can nurse 'around the clock'.

Summary

I hope this chapter has helped you to identify factors you might not have considered when applying for a nursing programme, and provided some useful information and guidance regarding such issues as gaining experience in a care setting, travel and childcare. Remember – nursing is not just a course at university. It will require 50 per cent of your time to be spent in practice settings, with all that that entails. But at the end of your training you will have an academic qualification in the form of a degree and a professional qualification, allowing you to register with the NMC and practise as a nurse.

Although the course is challenging and demanding, you will be successful if you plan ahead and prepare. By learning about expectations, placement areas and travel (as well as other things) you can be confident that you are fully prepared to undertake your nurse development. Planning, communication and time management will make things easier in most areas – both as a student and as a registered nurse. Good luck!

References

Bennis, W.G. (2009) *On Becoming a Leader*, 4th Edn. New York: Perseus.
Compassionate Care: www.england.nhs.uk/wp-content/uploads/2012/12/6c-a5-leaflet.pdf (accessed 16 July 2014).

Kane, A. and Gooding, C. (2009) *Reasonable Adjustments in Nursing and Midwifery: A Literature Review Undertaken on Behalf of the Nursing and Midwifery Council*. London: Nursing and Midwifery Council.

NHS Bursaries Unit (2010) *Help with Childcare Costs for NHS Students*. London: NHS Business Services Authority.

Nursing and Midwifery Council (2008) *Standards to Support Learning and Assessment in Practice*. London: Nursing and Midwifery Council.

Nursing and Midwifery Council (2010) *Standards for Pre-registration Nursing Education*. London: Nursing and Midwifery Council.

Nursing and Midwifery Council (2011) *Guidance on Professional Conduct for Nursing and Midwifery Students*. London: Nursing and Midwifery Council.

Nursing and Midwifery Council (2015) *The Code: Professional Standards of Practice and Behaviour for Nurses and Midwives*. London: Nursing and Midwifery Council.

Siviter, B. (2013) *Student Nurse Handbook: A Survival Guide*, 3rd Edn. Edinburgh: Bailliere Tindall.

Further reading

Clarke, L. and Hawkins, J. (2001) *Student Survival Guide: What to Expect and How to Handle it – Insider Advice on University Life*. Oxford: How To Books.

Useful web links

Interactive driving maps: www.bing.com/maps
NHS Bursary: www.nhsbsa.nhs.uk/studentdocuments
NHS Jobs: www.nhs.jobs.uk
Nursing and Midwifery Council: www.nmc-uk.org
Ofsted information about early years childcare: www.ofsted.gov.uk/early-years-and-childcare
Public transport information: www.traveline.info
Unistats: www.unistats.com
UCAS: www.ucas.ac.uk.

Chapter 13

Life during clinical practice placements

Trevor Parker, with Kate Wadley

The National Health Service (NHS) today is very different from the one I started working in almost 30 years ago. During this time I have worked in theatres, elderly care, and acute, renal and respiratory medicine – before moving into professional development and, for the past 14 years, student support. In this chapter I will discuss 'life' during clinical placements within an acute hospital setting, giving you a realistic view of what to expect and some coping strategies you may find helpful when you are on your clinical placements.

What is a clinical practice placement?

A clinical practice placement is where a nursing student applies their knowledge to practice, learns key skills and achieves the required competencies for registration.

Clinical placements are an essential part of any nursing degree programme across the UK. The Nursing and Midwifery Council (NMC) require nursing students to complete no less than 50 per cent of the programme in the clinical area (NMC 2010) which equates to 2300 hours during your three-year training programme.

Learning in the contextual setting of clinical practice enables students to confront many of the challenges and issues related to caring. Clinical practice is where lifelong learning is promoted and enhanced.

Research evidence suggests that practice education allows students to practise problem-solving skills, to observe and question the application of practice, and to gain insight into the reality of work and the pressures of the work environment (Alsop and Ryan 1996). In addition, having placements in a range of settings enables students to gain a comprehensive view of healthcare service delivery and helps to inform their future career choice. The Willis Commission (2012) recommends that practice and academic staff work together to help students relate theory to practice. It also highlights that patient-centred care should be the golden thread that runs through all pre-registration nurse education.

When on any clinical placement you will be given supervised opportunities to practise and develop the skills required to deliver healthcare. Box 13.1 shows just a sample of the activities during clinical placements.

There will always be a range of skills that you can or cannot do at certain points during your three-year programme of study. It is for the registered practitioner to determine:

(a) If a particular skill is suitable for you to undertake;
(b) If you have any previous knowledge or experience in this area;
(c) Does it require you to have direct supervision and/or guidance to ensure safe practice?

Box 13.1 Sample activities during clinical placements

- Direct care giving
- Observation of registered practitioners
- Visits to other wards/departments for specialist practitioners
- Directed student activities which require the student to access appropriate resources and policies, and analyse or evaluate them
- Workshops/teaching sessions/case presentations
- Clinical teaching and learning
- Collaborative working, e.g. meetings, case conferences
- Simulated scenarios/role play
- Reflective practice.

As a student, however, you have a responsibility for your own practice/competence and you should question what you are being asked to do. Nonetheless, the accountability for care rests with the registered practitioner and most will be governed by local hospital policy.

The complex nature of patients' needs requires nurses to work collaboratively with many other professionals and, as a result, you should experience placements that prepare you for this aspect of the role.

In addition to achieving your learning outcomes whilst on placement, staff will have other expectations of students (see Figure 13.1). As I am sure you can see, these

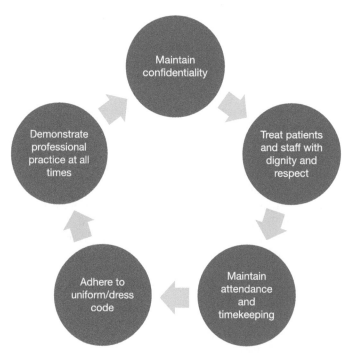

Figure 13.1 Expectations of students during clinical placements

expectations extend to all healthcare employees and form the bedrock of what we call 'professionalism'.

Whilst working in practice you will be required to demonstrate appropriate professional conduct at all times. During your clinical placements you will be 'supernumerary', i.e. not counted as part of the workforce, but there is anticipation that you will be involved in care delivery wherever your clinical placement is. I prefer the term 'participant observer', which means that you will observe but also take part in care delivery, as you cannot learn by observation alone.

Placement experiences will include providing nursing care to some of society's most vulnerable people – the elderly, the very young, those who are physically or mentally ill, and others who may have a physical or learning disability. Practice experiences build throughout the course and are the reason why the NMC places so much emphasis on the completion of practice hours.

Hospital placements

Regardless of which field of nursing you choose (except perhaps learning disabilities) you will be allocated a number of clinical placements in the hospital setting. During these placements you will care for patients suffering from acute and long-term illnesses and diseases. Chapters 4–7 have already provided you with an insight into the uniqueness of the different fields of nursing, so you can appreciate how hospital placements relate to clinical practice and clinical care. So, in a hospital setting you may find yourself supporting patients' recovery from illness or operation, by focusing on the needs of the patient rather than their illness or condition. You will undoubtedly experience healthcare professionals promoting good health and well-being through patient education, and of course you will usually find yourself working within a multidisciplinary team.

Gaining the trust and confidence of each patient is important, but it also extends to developing good relationships with the patient's relatives/carers as well. Patients may be admitted to hospital for surgery, for treatment of chronic or acute illnesses, to accident and

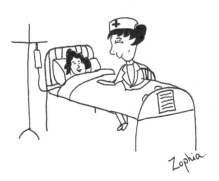

emergency with injuries, or simply attending an outpatient clinic or undergoing tests and assessments. Hospital placements therefore offer a wide scope of clinical experience for you to develop your knowledge and skills in order for you to successfully gain your NMC nursing registration.

For nurses delivering healthcare, whatever the setting, the central focus is always the individual patient and the provision of holistic care, coupled with the involvement of their family (and often close friends).

Working shifts

The reality of 24-hour healthcare delivery means that many healthcare workers are required to work a variety of shift patterns. Adapting to shift patterns (or changes in shift patterns) can be difficult. As humans we have a 24-hour body clock called a circadian rhythm. This rhythm is controlled by the brain and regulates how our bodies react to certain aspects of our lives – for example, the times we sleep, wake, eat, and our body temperature, pulse and blood pressure.

Adequate rest breaks within shifts are essential to prevent excessive tiredness and fatigue, and for maintaining your health and for refuelling when working in a physically demanding role. The Working Time Regulations state that when a shift lasts six hours or more, the worker is entitled to a minimum 20-minute rest break (RCN 2012a).

People require healthcare 24 hours a day, 7 days a week, 365 days of the year, in a variety of settings. The NMC requires students to experience the full range of clinical experiences, including the need to work outside of the traditional working week of Monday to Friday, 9 to 5. Therefore, you will be expected to work morning shifts, which start between 7 a.m. and 8 a.m., afternoon shifts, which can finish as late as 9.30 p.m., as well as night shifts, weekends and Bank Holidays.

Punctuality is essential when you are on placement, as being late sends the wrong (not professional) message, and you may miss out on information and learning opportunities.

Before you start a new clinical placement it is a really good idea to prepare by finding out some information about it. For example, you could use a range of resources including placement profiles, which can often be found on the university or hospital websites. Always try to read up on the speciality, and contact the placement area at least 5–10 days before starting the placement to discuss shift patterns, and arrange a pre-placement visit if possible.

Read any induction material available – most areas will have a welcome/student information pack. During your placement you will have initial, midway and final interviews with your mentor. So identify your strengths and weaknesses, and be prepared to discuss with your mentor how your learning outcomes can be achieved. Make sure you understand what is expected of you as a student. The NMC (2010a) guide for students will help, as will your university placement document.

Acute care

Acute nursing care is a general term for short-term hospital-based or emergency healthcare services. Acute illnesses are sudden in onset and can also go quickly, and in the middle – during treatment – can be quite severe. A stab wound, for example, is an acute problem which lasts until the wound heals. This pattern of care is often only necessary for a short time, unlike chronic or continuing care.

On an acute clinical placement you will have the chance to see the treatment of patients with serious conditions. This could be through a placement like A&E, where you will learn how to react quickly, an intensive care unit, an acute medical or surgical ward, or indeed in an acute psychiatric unit.

During your placement you will very quickly come to realise that nursing is a demanding vocation which requires hard work, commitment, and the ability to problem solve, work independently and contribute to care as part of a team. You will be required to have an understanding of a range of conditions that affect patients and their families or carers. It is important that you are able to recognise how illness affects patients both physically and psychologically.

Continuing care

Continuing care nursing is provided over an extended period of time to meet physical or mental health needs that have arisen as a result of disability, an accident or long-term illness. Continuing care also refers to patients who require ongoing care and care across different environments/multiple agencies. It is therefore good to get to know the nursing care needs of the patients with chronic illness.

The aim of continuing care is to provide appropriate long-term support, promote independence, prevent physical and mental deterioration and maximise a person's health and quality of life. This type of placement will enhance your knowledge in the holistic care of individuals with chronic illness, and improve your understanding of disease causation.

At times it can feel as though you are only really doing bed-baths, but remember when helping someone with their daily hygiene needs, you can learn some interesting life history! It can be quite a satisfying experience giving someone a bath, though it may not seem the most remarkable or glamorous of events for the majority of nurses/students. Think of a patient who suffers from a chronic condition, who has not been able to have a bath for some time, perhaps as a result of a disability/condition. In assisting them to have a bath you could receive the warmest gratitude – and that can be really rewarding and make you feel so good!

You will get to see progress as patients gradually get better or more mobile; you will notice small but significant changes, which gives great satisfaction. Real learning is done on placement and it should be seen as a great opportunity to chat through the theory you've learned at university and relate to what things work in practice. This is sometimes referred to as theory-related or evidence-based practice, so you can start to understand how and why things are done the way they are.

Support during clinical practice placements

The NMC (2008) requires that students are continually assessed in practice. Whilst on placement you will be supervised by a mentor – a registered nurse who has successfully completed an approved 'preparation for mentorship' programme. Mentors are accountable for the decisions made about a student's competence (NMC 2008). It is therefore necessary to have sufficient skilled, knowledgeable practitioners within placement areas who can take on the role of a mentor.

The pace of work on clinical placements can seem quite fast when you are not used to it or when you are first starting out. Indeed it can seem that the wards are understaffed – which means of course that students can feel that they are undervalued or even in the way of the busy nurses. What is important is that, however busy your clinical placement is, time should be allocated to learning alongside your mentor so that you gain as much experience as possible during your allocated time with them.

Sometimes you may feel out of your depth. It is all very new – and you have an assignment or an exam to study for in the midst of all this. And the clinical placement experience you get can vary from the other students in your group. This all makes for a very stressful time and may leave you wondering 'What am I doing this for?'

One of the biggest concerns students express whilst on their clinical placement is being at a loose end. Students often express this through statements such as, 'I don't know what to do', 'I feel like a spare part', 'I stand around quite often with my hands in my pockets' and 'I don't want to look like I haven't got anything to do'. So what do you do when you haven't got a specific task or duty to perform? What you will be able to do will depend on the stage of your training. As a first-year student you may not be able to do very much, unless under direct supervision, so looking in the patient's notes or speaking to the patient/relative is probably your best option. This will aid your learning about health and illness and its impact on the patient's life/lifestyle. It can also help you in building relationships and improve your communication skills.

Your first clinical shift can be frightening, and you may feel like you are being thrown into the deep end of the swimming pool without any visible lifesavers. You do not know where any equipment is, where you can leave your belongings/valuables, where the sluice is, where to wash your hands, where the patient charts are kept, what you are supposed to document, etc. Do not fret – you are not alone!

Thankfully you will not be the only one feeling like this within your group – others will be feeling just the same. What do you do? Remember, each clinical placement will have its own 'culture', norms and standard ways to do things that have been created by members of the area. This type of disoriented feeling can occur with every new placement, and it is absolutely normal. With each placement you may find it easier to adapt to the different cultures. This is what Waters (2001) calls 'enculturation', the process by which students are inducted and adopt their professional culture.

Here are some tips that might help with orienting into a new placement area. Become familiar with any emergency equipment – where to find it, which button you should press for emergencies. Determine the layout of the placement, identify a friendly face, and relax. As you settle into the placement and after meeting the staff and having handover you can start to find out what equipment is most often used, and then take some time to figure out quickly how things work.

Even on the first day, don't be afraid to ask questions. A smile, eye contact and just openness to talk will help you to settle, and will demonstrate your desire and enthusiasm to become part of the team and learn from experts. And remember your mentor is there to help and support you – and indeed you will realise what a great resource the whole team are.

Get your essential care sorted and spend time with the healthcare assistants who you will realise are invaluable. Remember your limitations – don't do things you have not been taught at university. Use your placements to understand the workings of that particular area and delivering care, such as personal hygiene, bed changing, observations. These things are vital and you are ensuring they don't get missed out. Don't worry if your fellow students came back from their placement bragging about things they had got to do. All placements are different and your time will come.

Undertake background reading while on placement. Make the most of feedback given and ask questions – even if you think they are stupid – especially if you come across something you don't understand or are unsure of. Always show a genuine interest in what your nursing mentor has to say. I have been a mentor many times and nothing is worse than having a student who is uninterested or does not pay attention. Being attentive shows the mentor that you want to learn from them and if you don't demonstrate this they are less likely to want to help you.

There will be times when you might feel brushed off, or told to find the answer yourself. Don't be offended – this will happen and the nurses you shadow don't mean to ignore you. Instead, try to find the answer through other resources: internet, library, other students, healthcare assistants or other nurses. Be persistent, you are there to learn, and it is for your patients' safety that you ask. At the same time, you have to use your judgement as to whether there is information you should know before going into the placement.

No matter what placement you are in, remember that all patients and families are unique, with individual needs. It is your responsibility to ensure their needs are made known and being addressed (i.e. patient-/family-centred). Whilst on placement, if a procedure is being done – ask to observe! With things such as operations, angiograms or lumbar punctures, you would not get the opportunity as a registered nurse, and it can help you understand what the procedure actually involves when explaining it to patients. This will also enable you to understand a patient's journey.

Make sure you know *exactly* what you're doing. If you are being asked to carry out a procedure for the first time – even if you've done it in university – *make sure* you are supervised, and know how to carry it out. It is OK to make mistakes – as long as you are not endangering life or trying to do things that you should not be for your stage of training. If you make a mistake, don't beat yourself up, but learn from it instead. If you mess up it is easy to feel you have let people down – but you are there to learn! Finally, your mentor is there to help you, and you will also have a personal tutor allocated to support you, so if you need help in any aspect of your training don't hesitate to ask.

Coping with disabilities/reasonable adjustments

Not every student with a disability will require additional support whilst on their practice placements. To establish if the student requires any additional support, the disability contact within the university will review the student's individual learning plan/assessment, formulated when the student started the programme. Before going out on placement, this will be reviewed and, if necessary, adjusted to identify any particular needs the student may have in relation to that placement. This review will be undertaken with the student, and a joint decision made about the best way to provide support for the student.

Reasonable adjustments to address these actual/potential challenges are usually recommended. Implementing these adjustments will enable the student to experience a meaningful and engaging placement. The student will still be required to meet the outcomes and proficiency statements specified in the practical assessment document.

Students need to be mindful that it is their responsibility to ensure that practice staff are made aware of the requirements they may have in line with their disability, in order to facilitate reasonable adjustments.

Student nurse testimonials

I am always nervous when I first start a new placement. On my first placement on an elderly female ward, I was completely new to healthcare and didn't really know what to expect. I loved it right from my first day. After a few days, when I had got to know the staff and ward routine, I started to feel like part of the team.

The most daunting part of starting to placement for me was delivering personal care to patients. I quickly realised how much of a valuable skill it is. You get to talk to the patient, find out how they are feeling and their concerns but you are also able to assess them, noting things such as their skin integrity and mobility. I found the healthcare assistants invaluable in my learning. They really are an integral part of the team. It was through them that I learned a lot of skills, like how to deliver personal care, how to fill in the bedside paperwork and where everything is!

I have got on with all my mentors. It can be hard sometimes on busy areas to get time with them to learn, but I quickly got into the knack of knowing what I needed to learn and chasing them round the ward to observe certain skills. I find having a pocket notebook essential. If I come across something I do not know, I note it down and look it up properly when I get home. There is always something you need to write down, be it a set of observations or even a patient's preference for tea or coffee. You don't always have patients' paperwork to hand.

The patients are what I love most about placements. When patients are in hospital for weeks, you can really get to know them and miss them when they go home. It is so rewarding to see patients making progress and knowing that you have helped in that journey.

Emma Broome BSc Nursing (Adult)

Seeing that smile on the face of a child who is recovering, or a critically ill child whose health is improving, can give you so much job satisfaction. Caring for someone who is not your own seems hard but it takes certain people to do it. I have done it, and I didn't realise the joy from doing so until I started nursing. It is as if you are that ray of light for a child – without them even being able to express their needs, you understand. Without even realising, you are supporting the whole family because it all comes hand in hand. A professional, a teacher, an advocate, a carer . . . Best profession I could ever be in.

Rachel Droach BSc Nursing (Child)

I spent a long time working within the criminal justice system and I wanted to work in forensic mental health. But since starting and having a variety of placements I have become passionate about mental health on a level I never felt possible, and I can't quite believe that my mind changes daily on where I want to work when I qualify. When we started, we were told we were privileged to be mental health nurses, and my initial thoughts were 'and they thought I was fluffy'. But now I see it and now I get it, and that sense of pride and achievement I have felt working with the patients I have in such a short space of time is something I hadn't felt in the several years I had poured into my last career.

Gemma Macken BSc Nursing (Mental Health)

Being a child's nurse is an amazing position to be in, as I feel I have made a difference in a child's life, no matter how small. The trust that is built and the responsibility shared with the parents is never forgotten. I feel I am in a special position to bring hope and courage for the whole family and be the shoulder for them to cry on.

Amira Mohamed BSc Nursing (Child)

Community placements

Community nursing has changed dramatically over the last decade, following the UK-wide priority shift of moving patient care out of the acute hospitals and into the community. In order to manage this shift of care, the community workforces are required to be highly skilled in many areas and are considered to be the mainstay of locally delivered healthcare across the UK (RCN 2010). To support this, nursing care and elements of social care are now delivered by multi-professionals who make up a community team to provide holistic care in the patient's home.

The work of nurses in the community encompasses the promotion of health, healing, growth and development, as well as the prevention and treatment of disease, illness, injury and disability (Royal College of Nursing 2010, 2012b).

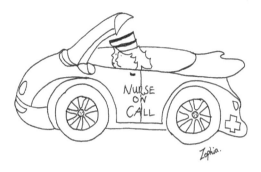

Community nursing comes into two fields – one focused on children, young people and their families, the other focused on adults and older adults. Additionally, where appropriate, community nursing focuses support on generalist health services.

In the past, student nurses were allocated to community placements with a district nursing team or a health-visiting team, dependent on the branch of nursing undertaken, but now with many professionals providing specialist care for patients in the community, a placement could be with a range of professionals. Every effort is taken to provide a period, of from one or two days up to two weeks if possible, to allow the student to observe a specialist professional as part of a package of care provided by a multi-professional team. Community teams have access to the full range of physical and mental health capacity and capability needs to deliver holistic care.

Advancements in medical and health technology have enabled the population to live longer, and some patients will need complex care interventions, requiring the workforce to be highly skilled. The skill mix of practitioners within teams is very varied. Teams may include district nurses, health visitors, school nurses, allied health professionals (such as occupational therapists, physiotherapists, speech and language, etc.) and social care workers such as community healthcare co-ordinators and social workers.

In some community healthcare trusts there are community hospitals and rehabilitation services to support respite care (to enable everyday carers to have a break from caring for loved ones). There are also teams in the community named 'rapid response teams' who provide a package of care for a short-term period to allow a patient to stay at home rather than be admitted to a hospital.

District nurses, health visitors and school nurses are qualified nurses who have undertaken a further graduate specialist practitioner programme. When these practitioners undertake the course they are supported by 'practice teachers' who assess and sign off their practice. A typical team led by district nurses is supported by registered nurses who are community staff nurses and healthcare assistants and support staff. Health visitor teams also have community nurses and nursery nurses, plus support workers who deliver child-centred care. School nurses have community staff nurses and support workers to assist with health education sessions and childhood immunisation in schools.

There is uniqueness in the community as practitioners work alone. Therefore every student works on a one-to-one basis with their allocated registered mentor. You will travel around the city in the mentor's car unless they have other travel arrangements (but you will be advised of the travel arrangements when you contact the team two weeks before placement). Students are not expected to use their own transport between patient visits as they cannot claim any travelling expenses. The arrangements to meet with your identified mentor are usually at the medical centre/health centre, school or residential centre.

There will be opportunities whilst on placement to work, not only with your mentor, but with other members of the multi-disciplinary team. Each team will have a 'menu of alternative learning experience' and there may be an opportunity to spend a day with the practice nurse in a GP surgery, community diabetes team, long-term conditions team or coroner's court, for example. Students are encouraged to arrange alternative experiences in which they are interested.

As communities are geographically widespread it would be impossible to have all students in one area for induction days. Therefore there are local inductions within placement teams. Some community NHS trusts have an electronic student 'hub' website for students to access. This usually includes information regarding the trust and what services are available, student quizzes, reading lists, etc. (though this will vary from organisation to organisation).

Community care is mainly carried out in a patient's home and the professional and student are the patient's guests. Respect of the patient's property is therefore to be adhered to at all times. Some homes may not be like your own, but you should never display any signs of displeasure or amazement at a home – you should remain non-judgemental and impartial.

Care can also be delivered in elderly care day centres, residential homes, GP practices, schools, special schools, prisons, learning-disability shared homes and centres, and identified areas for outreach services, such as the homeless and travelling families.

Community nursing care is delivered 24 hours a day. There are shift patterns: perhaps 8–6 or 9–5 for day staff, and 5–10 for evening staff, followed by provision of a city night service. There are also other agencies providing care out of hours – for example, Macmillan or Marie Curie services, caring for terminally ill people. There are also voluntary services who 'sit' with patients day or night to assist carers, or to allow carers to have a night's rest.

There will be a wide range of clinical and managerial skills that you may be able to take part in or observe in various placements. Box 13.2 lists some of the most common clinical skills you may encounter whilst on community placements.

There are also nurse-led and other professional clinics where patients are monitored, treated and discharged solely by the expert knowledge and experience of the practitioner. There are also many practitioners who are 'nurse prescribers' and this skill helps with the process of enabling nursing care to commence effectively and efficiently.

Technological developments are assisting healthcare professionals. Some district nursing teams are currently using mobile working devices. These enable all paperwork to be electronically recorded immediately at the assessment of patients' needs. This allows more

---

Box 13.2 Common community clinical skills

- Prompting medication administration
- Administering insulin and other injections
- Short- and long-term wound care, with additional knowledge of tissue viability
- Palliative care
- Intravenous (IV) therapy
- Male/female urethral catheterisation
- Tracheostomy care
- Continence assessment
- Blood glucose monitoring
- Nasogastric or gastrostomy tube feeding.

Box 13.3 Examples of community placements

- Patients' own homes
- Residential care homes
- Prisons
- Day care centres
- Special schools
- Community nursing teams
- Health visitors
- Satellite haemodialysis units
- Outreach services.

---

time for face-to-face patient care and reduces the need for paper clinical records and duplicate data entry.

Community placements are varied and Box 13.3 provides some examples.

Summary

Nursing offers a wide variety of experiences and placements to support you and enable you to relate your theory to practice. Support in practice is available from a variety of different practitioners – and the university, as well.

Hopefully this chapter has provided you with a good insight as to what life in clinical placements can be like, and given you some useful coping strategies to aid your learning and assist you to get the most out of your clinical placements.

References

Alsop, A.E. and Ryan, S.E. (1996) *Making the Most of Fieldwork Education: A Practical Approach.* Andover: Cengage Learning EMEA.

Department of Health (2013) *Care in Local Communities: A New Vision and Model for District Nursing.* London: DH.

Nursing and Midwifery Council (2008) *Standards to Support Learning and Assessment in Practice.* London: Nursing and Midwifery Council.

Nursing and Midwifery Council (2010) *Standards for Pre-registration Nursing Education.* London: Nursing and Midwifery Council.

Nursing and Midwifery Council (2011) *Guidance on Professional Conduct for Nursing and Midwifery Students.* London: Nursing and Midwifery Council.

Reading, S. and Webster, B. (2013) *Achieving Competencies for Nursing Practice: A Handbook for Student Nurses.* Maidenhead: McGraw Hill/Open University Press.

Royal College of Nursing (2008) *Nursing our Future: An RCN Study into the Challenges Facing Today's Nursing Students in the UK.* London: RCN Publishing.

Royal College of Nursing (2010) *Pillars of the Community: The RCN's UK Position on the Development of the Registered Nursing Workforce in the Community.* London: RCN Publishing.

Royal College of Nursing (2012a) *A Shift in the Right Direction.* London: RCN Publishing, www.rcn.org.uk/publications (accessed 6 March 2014).

Royal College of Nursing (2012b) *The Community Nursing Workforce in England*. London: RCN Publishing.

Waters, B. (2001) Radical action for radical plans. *The British Journal of Occupational Therapy* 64(ii): 577–578.

Willis (2012) *Quality with Compassion: The Future of Nursing Education (Report of the Willis Commission on Nursing Education)*. London: RCN Publishing.

Further reading

Boyd, V. and McKendry, S. (2012) *Getting Ready for Your Nursing Degree: The StudySMART Guide to Learning at University*. Harlow: Pearson.

Levett-Jones, T. and Bourgeois, S. (2009) *The Clinical Placement: A Nursing Survival Guide*, 2nd Edn. London: Bailliere Tindall.

Richards, A. and Edwards, S.L. (2012) *A Nurse's Survival Guide to the Ward*, 3rd Edn. Edinburgh: Churchill Livingstone.

Royal College of Nursing (2006) *Helping Students Get the Best from Their Practice Placements*. London: RCN Publishing.

Siviter, B. (2013) *The Student Nurse Handbook: A Survival Guide*, 3rd Edn. Edinburgh: Bailliere Tindall.

Useful web links

Nursing and Midwifery Council: www.nmc-uk.org
Nursing Times: http://info.nursingtimes.net/student
Nursing Standard: www.nursing-standard-journal.co.uk
Royal College of Nursing: www.rcn.org.uk.

Chapter 14

Stresses of being a student nurse

Cathy Poole

Starting your nursing programme will be one of the most amazing – and perhaps one of the most stressful and most nerve-racking – times of your life. Being well prepared and knowing what to expect will help you to deal with the stresses ahead of you.

When you arrive at your chosen university for the first time it is likely to be one of those challenging life events which you can only have imagined before! Reality is about to set in and you will experience a myriad of feelings – some good, some not so good – and many which will leave a lasting impression on you. I hope this chapter can help you to have some insight into the stresses you may encounter during your three-year programme, and to have an awareness of how to deal with these stresses. Students who have already experienced what you are about to experience have offered some personal insights into how they have coped and developed the strength to be successful.

Moving away from home

For many student nurses, starting a three-year nursing programme includes moving away from home for the very first time. This in itself can be a daunting prospect. If you have done your research and visited the campus accommodation during open days then hopefully you will have a good idea of what to expect from the accommodation and, importantly, what

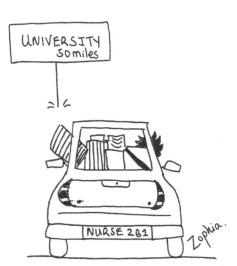

the monthly costs will be. Most student nurses live in halls of residence during their first year. This is beneficial as you will quickly get to know people who are undertaking a variety of degree studies and it will certainly help you to navigate your way around the university campus. Knowing what to expect can really help to reduce your stress (and that of your family). So knowing what the halls consist of, what each room is equipped with, what the laundry facilities are like and whether they are coin-operated or not and, importantly, what the security around the campus is like, will all help you to settle in.

Suddenly becoming self-sufficient when it comes to shopping for food, cooking, washing and ironing can come as a bit of a shock, so

---

Box 14.1 Stresses of moving away from home

Locational

- Not familiar with the local area
- Navigating new public transport timetables
- Getting to clinical placements on time
- Safety/security

Personal

- Money worries
- Feeling homesick
- Cooking for yourself
- Sticking to a budget
- Washing and ironing
- Making new friends
- Personal safety
- Feeling isolated
- Coping with disabilities.

---

get some practice before you leave home. Box 14.1 shows some of the common stresses linked to being away from home.

The best way to cope with these potential stressors is linked to the aspects we discussed in Chapter 9 about your initial research during your application process and about making the most of university open days. Remember you will not be the only new student who feels stressed at this stage, so find out who the people are who you are sharing accommodation with and get involved with student life early. Make the most of what Freshers' Week has to offer and explore your new environment.

Money matters

One of the biggest worries that all students have is linked to money – or should I say the lack of it! In Chapter 9 we outlined the bursary scheme available for student nurses and, of course, the fact that university fees are paid for you. Money saved in advance of starting your programme can be a good buffer and will help you to set a budget. So while you are waiting to start your course, try to be creative in how you build up your savings.

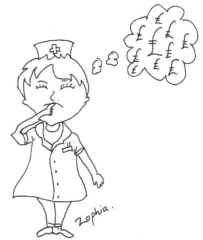

Many student nurses continue to have or find part-time jobs during their three-year nurse training programmes. Whilst this may be of great assistance in keeping you on financial track remember it must never impact negatively on your ability to be successful in your academic studies and clinical placement commitments. One thing I often say to student nurses is: 'You only have three years of austerity . . . with a professional lifetime of earning potential ahead of you.'

I know of many students who luckily have some financial help from their families during their studies. I also know that some students find it very difficult to manage their own finances. Do not despair, as all universities have departments within their student support services who are able to offer expert advice linked to money matters and, in some instances, they will be able to point you in the direction of additional financial support. My advice is to apply for your bursary and student loan as soon as possible, and if money issues are becoming a real stress for you ask for help early – talk to your tutors, student services and your family.

On the RCN student website (www.rcn.org.uk/development/students) you will be able to find some good advice linked to your bursary, benefits, housing and money matters – and, importantly, they offer some top tips on managing your finances.

Combining academic and clinical learning

The importance of combining academic studies (theory) with clinical learning (practice) cannot be over-emphasised. Theory and practice are inextricably linked and, as discussed in Chapters 12 and 13, the time spent on these two elements is split equally during your three-year programme (NMC 2010).

Chapter 13 provided you with some sound information which will hopefully assist you in dealing with the stresses associated with your clinical placements. What I would say is that if any of the clinical situations you find yourself in are overwhelming, you should talk them through as soon as possible with your mentor or university personal tutor. Remember – a problem shared is a problem halved! Your mentors and the university tutors will have had previous experience of dealing with stressful clinical scenarios faced by students and they will be more than happy to help you deal with them.

Meeting academic deadlines

In my experience, student nurses are far more likely to feel stressed about their academic studies than their clinical placements. A good tip is to get an academic diary and write down all your assignment deadlines, portfolio requirements, reflective accounts, key hand-in dates, numeracy tests, exam dates, etc. Some students put a year planner up on their wall, with all the key dates on, as a constant reminder to help them keep on track, and taking great pleasure in ticking them off as they make progress through their training. Many universities offer examination support/revision classes/one-to-one tutorials and also academic study skills classes. If you have any doubts about your study skills or ability to study at the next level, make use of all the help which is on offer.

When you get assignments or examination results back it is really good practice to take note of the feedback provided by the tutors, as they will most likely have made some suggestions as to how you can make improvements for your next piece of work. This is particularly relevant if you do not pass an assessment. If this happens, seek help early and make the most of revision classes. And make sure that you know when the next resubmission date is.

Box 14.2 Useful tips to help reduce the stress of meeting academic deadlines

- Know what the assessment is about
- Start your research early
- Make the most of tutorials
- Use recommended reading lists
- Plan a revision timetable for examinations
- Ask for help early – don't leave it until the last minute
- Make sure you understand the academic jargon
- Make friends with the recommended university referencing tool
- Look after yourself and eat healthily
- Make time for breaks and have some fun
- Build a support network
- Get an academic diary
- Make use of a wall planner
- Be realistic about the time it takes to write essays
- Find a balance between work, rest and play
- Get to know your university library
- Know when/how to request an extension to a deadline
- Try not to leave things until the last minute
- Make use of all the available learning resources
- Learn how to respond to constructive criticism
- Keep in touch with your tutors

You will need to develop your own way of keeping on top of your academic workload. Do not get stressed by seeing others who seem to glide through their academic assessments – remember to think about yourself and develop coping strategies that help you.

Most lecturers know of students who leave things until the last minute, apparently relaxed. They also know of students who find academic assessment deadlines stressful, even when they plan ahead methodically, and some students who find academic deadlines and personal academic skills so stressful that they become unwell. Box 14.2 shows some useful tips which might help to prevent these stresses. Whilst this list is not exhaustive, hopefully it will give you some ideas to take with you to university.

Research and referencing skills

Many student nurses find it stressful getting to grips with various things – research terminology, how to undertake a literature search and navigate their way around recommended search engines, how to critically analyse research to support their arguments in assignments, and then (if that wasn't stressful enough) how to correctly apply the recommended university referencing tool, perhaps Harvard or Vancouver!

All universities offer support in this area because they know that research skills and referencing skills are not normally strengths that new student nurses bring with them. So avail yourself of all the help you can get, whether that is through pre-arranged study skills sessions, group tutorials, referencing workshops, online support or utilising university referencing tools. One of the best ways I know of trying to understand how to reference correctly and use critical analysis is by reading, reading and more reading of research papers. That way you can see the styles of academic writing and how Harvard or Vancouver referencing is applied, as well as gaining knowledge of the subject matter.

One of the things you must be particularly mindful of is that you understand the notion of cheating and plagiarism. Cheating can be described as a situation whereby a student has tried to gain unfair advantage during an exam or assessment. This may involve the student breaching the university's examination/assessment conduct rules. Plagiarism, on the other hand, is defined as an attempt by the student to try to pass off the work of somebody else as their own. Sometimes a student's lack of referencing skills culminates in unintentional plagiarism – another reason to get all the help you can to develop your referencing knowledge and skills. All universities take cheating and plagiarism extremely seriously. They investigate any suspicion robustly and place sanctions on students if their suspicions are well founded. In some instances students can be removed from their programmes of study. So make sure you really understand how to avoid cheating and plagiarism. It is not worth the stress of getting caught. Most universities will provide some very clear advice on how to have a cheating-free and plagiarism-free approach to your studies, so take all the advice you can get. It is free and will stand you in good stead.

Coping with disabilities

Coming to university with identified disabilities may be a daunting prospect. However all universities have excellent systems and processes in place which are designed to ensure that disabilities do not pose barriers for any students, regardless of the programme being studied.

Declaration of any disabilities early in your application process will pay dividends, as many universities will begin to assess individual needs in advance of your university start date. This ensures that everything is in place in readiness for the start of your three-year course, which will really help to reduce the stress associated with coping with a disability in a new environment. UCAS offer some good disability advice which includes a short video which will help allay any worries you might have concerning disabilities.

Figure 14.1 provides an overview of the range of some of the services offered by university disabilities services.

Of particular relevance for students with disabilities is their potential to access disabled student allowances (DSA). As nursing programmes are funded by the NHS, you will automatically be sent a DSA1 form to apply for this allowance – but only if you declare your disability on your NHS bursary application form. Early declaration will remove this from your worry list.

Sometimes students contact university disability services because they are struggling with their academic studies and have a feeling that they may have an undiagnosed disability, such as dyslexia, for example. Disability services have the right tools in place to support and fully assess students who have dyslexia, as well as other learning difficulties. Again the message here is contact the experts early as there may be specific support you could be offered – for example assistive technology. Assistive technologies are those which provide dyslexia-friendly software, such as Dictaphones or voice-recognition features. McPheat (2014) provides an overview of the experiences of nursing students who have dyslexia and the impact it potentially has during their experiences in clinical practice.

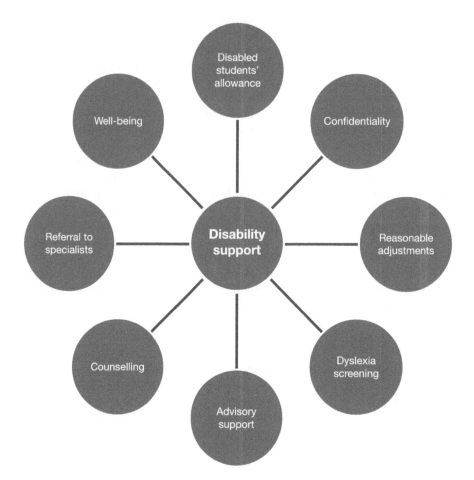

Figure 14.1 Sample range of services offered by university disability services

Of particular importance for students with disabilities is the notion of 'reasonable adjustments'. As explained earlier, there are statutory requirements, the Equality Act in England, Wales and Scotland, and the Disability Discrimination Act in Northern Ireland, which set the statutory principles to make sure that every effort is made to accommodate students with disabilities and that optimum support is provided.

Student nurse testimonials

The following student testimonials outline the stresses of being a student nurse and offer some personal insights on how to cope and build resilience.

I previously had a career in banking for five years and found working in a sales environment unrewarding and unsatisfying. I decided I wanted a career where I could make a real difference to people's lives. My Mum's personal battle with depression was what initially got me interested in mental health and it was then that I decided to take a new direction in life and return to university to study to become a mental health nurse.

I found returning to university as a mature student difficult at first. It had been six years since I was last in education and I initially struggled with the academic work. Writing assignments again was almost an alien concept to me, especially as my knowledge on nursing was limited due to me having no previous experience of working in mental health. My first placement allowed me to start building on this experience but also proved challenging as unforeseen circumstances meant my mentor changed three times. This proved to be a stressful time for me, but it was at this point that I started to use reflection as a tool, which in turn helped to manage my stress.

I started to reflect on my placement on a daily basis so I could make sense of what was happening on my shifts and how I was honestly feeling about these particular events. This helped to facilitate my learning by allowing me to consider what I learnt from an event and how I could do things differently next time. This allowed me to gain a more balanced perspective and reduce my stress levels as a result. It also taught me to not be so hard on myself if I made any mistakes because these mistakes were pointing out what areas I needed to improve on.

I then started to use reflection as a way of improving on my academic work. Reflecting on my first year, I could see that I didn't manage my time very well when it came to writing my assignments and this put me under much stress when I had deadlines looming. From this reflection I learnt that I needed to plan my time more effectively in my second year. As a result of this, in my second year I was less stressed, achieved higher grades and had more free time to relax.

Changing careers was a daunting choice for me to make, but on reflection I know it was the right choice to make. Reflection has allowed me to manage my stressors as a student nurse and I am confident that it will continue to help me to manage the stressors I encounter as I move throughout my career as a qualified nurse.

Steven Grainger
2nd year mental health student nurse
Birmingham City University

Throughout my two and a half years of being a student nurse I have had a lot of ups and many downs. There are many, many challenges that I have faced as a student nurse but these challenges are what keeps me going and what contributes to the exciting career that I have chosen to pursue.

Placements are what everyone worries about, and indeed I have faced many challenges during my clinical placements, both in hospital and in the community. I find it hard, having started a new placement, that when I have just got to know everyone, just got into the work routine, just started to understand what was going on! and just started to feel like I belong, when it's time to leave. Just like that. And then of course, start it all over again a few months later in the next placement.

I guess this is just something that you have to put up with as a student, but I think that being adaptable and showing enthusiasm helps in settling in quickly in order to get the most out of the short placements.

The other major stress of being a student is fitting in the academic work, placement, revision, practising clinical skills, reading and researching, and essay writing, all whilst trying to have some sort of social life! There have been times throughout my training that I have had so many things going on, both at uni and in my personal life, and have become overwhelmed, thinking 'How am I going to get through this?'

One thing that helped me was to have my eye on the end goal. So I had to keep reminding myself (or have other people reminding me!) what all this was for, and remembering why I want to be a nurse. This usually gets me back on track and able to focus. I also make sure that I have some sort of timetable or study planner, especially when there are lots of deadlines coming up. This helps to organise my time effectively, and having a plan written down helps make things clearer, so it's not going round and round in my head.

Nursing also comes with a load of emotional stresses. I deal with this by talking about things that are worrying me with someone close to me. Whether it be something that I've experienced on placement or getting stressed with an essay, I often call my parents or a close friend. This allows me to talk it through with someone outside the situation and also gain another perspective on things.

I think it's very important, as a student nurse, to remember to take time out of your busy workload and do something for yourself or something that you enjoy. Just taking a short walk in the park or reading a trashy book helps me to switch off and clear my mind, and be ready to face the next challenge!

Becky Fleming
3rd year adult student nurse
Kingston University

I am a third-year BSc (Hons) Child Nursing student at the University of Brighton. The end is rapidly approaching, and as I get nostalgic I have looked back over my training to explore the stresses I faced and how I coped.

It can be difficult to adjust to two roles: being a student and being a nursing student. These can be conflicting concepts; your timetable won't match your flatmates', and having to be up for placement when they come home from clubs can be awkward. Build a good relationship with your housemates; respect each other's needs. Tell them your shifts so they know which nights to sleep at another friend's house, or just go out together when you don't have placement. Your responsibilities must take priority, but allowing yourself time to relax is also important.

Placements are, understandably, a huge source of stress. What if my mentor doesn't like me? How do I adjust to diverse environments and make a good impression? Keep a log of shifts; you'll be surprised how much even a quiet night teaches you. Particularly at the beginning of a placement, you can feel rather 'in the way'. Be proactive: if you don't know something, get involved and ask questions. Never disrespect or undermine your mentor, but take note of the nurses who like to teach. Make the most of opportunities and do any task you can. Talk to your patients. Having the flexibility of a student is something many nurses wish they had, and often patients/parents tell me they just want someone to talk to. This is vital to your learning and the holistic care we can offer.

As with most students, money is an issue. With long terms you will need longer tenancies and you won't be able to get a long summer job. Figure out a budget: add up your necessities, add on some extra for having fun, and stick to it. An unnecessary bargain is still not a saving. I must say, the pound shop quickly became my best friend.

Being in the first cohort, I found the new degree programme was misunderstood by the media, public and even some colleagues. We were taught a lot about taking up the

NHS baton, being the caring, innovative and skilled professionals of the future . . . yet I met a lot of negativity. Remember: bad press makes good news. The NHS is not perfect, but I often go home astounded at the committed, compassionate and hardworking individuals I have the honour of working alongside. There are positive patient experiences every day and hundreds of unsung heroes. Let your actions change the 'too posh to wash' preconceptions.

Your personal and professional lives will affect each other. Situations at home affect how you react, and you sometimes feel like you've taken on all the emotion of patients and their relatives. Student services at university are a lifeline for financial advice, counselling, or support for extra educational needs. Your lecturers were all student nurses once – seek their understanding and advice. Make friends with the other student nurses; you will go through a lot together. I find the gym helps clear my mind, and have found unmatchable support and peace through a local church. Build a network; find a hobby or society to get stuck in to.

Although it sounds like my training was difficult, I have absolutely loved it. I have grown so much as an individual, met inspirational people and am excited to embark on my career. I wish you all the best in your training.

Megan Martin
3rd year child nursing student
University of Brighton

Summary

Nursing degrees are not designed to be easy. You are embarking on a professional career which brings big responsibility, commitment and often stressful work-related situations – and your training therefore needs to prepare you for this. You need to focus on your end result, give your best, take care of yourself, manage your time and, most important of all, make use of all the academic and clinical resources and advice available to you.

References

McPheat, C. (2014) Experience of nursing students with dyslexia on clinical placement. *Nursing Standard* 28(41): 44–49.

Nursing and Midwifery Council (2010) *Standards for Pre-Registration Nursing Education*. London: Nursing and Midwifery Council.

Further reading

Boyd, V. and McKendry, S. (2012) *Getting Ready for Your Nursing Degree: The StudySMART Guide to Learning at University*. Harlow: Pearson.

Elcock, K. (2012) *Getting into Nursing*. London: Sage.

Pike, C. (2013) *The Hungry Student Cookbook*. London: Quercus Editions.

Useful web links

Essex University (plagiarism and how to avoid it): www.essex.ac.uk/myskills/Plagiarism_and_how_to_avoid_it.pdf

Jamie Oliver's student recipes: www.jamieoliver.com/recipes/category/course/cheap-cheerful

Royal College of Nursing (Student Money Smart): www.rcn.org.uk_data/assets/pdf_file/0004/444802/RCN_Money_Smart_Full_PDF_v5.pdf

Royal College of Nursing for Students: www.rcn.org.uk/development/students

Student Nursing Times: http://info.nursingtimes.net/student-nursing-times

Student recipes on a tight budget: www.studentcook.co.uk

UCAS (students with disabilities): www.ucas.com/how-it-all-works/explore-your-options/individual-needs/students-disabilities.

Part 5

Beyond nurse training

Chapter 15

Employability

Ruth Lawton

Jobs!
Jobs?
Jobs ☺
Question: Where do you start?
Answer: Here

Whether you are reading this book because you are investigating the possibilities of nursing as a profession, or you are thinking about changing direction, or maybe you are approaching the end of your nurse training or even returning to the nursing profession – wherever you are in your working life – you need to be managing your career, keeping one step ahead of yourself to ensure that you are open to opportunities, possibilities and that you are *employable!*

Employability is not about getting a job – it is about managing our working lives. Before we retire we might be working for 40 or 50 years, and in that time we are likely to change jobs many times and even change career completely more than once. In the twenty-first century we no longer talk about a job for life, we talk about 'careers' and 'managing change' – particularly in the health services sector, where there is constant modernisation to improve effectiveness and efficiency. Employability is about valuing and recognising all of your experiences and how they are relevant for your current and future career.

Change happens at the big-picture level in terms of how 'health' is funded, managed and delivered; and it also happens at the level of nursing and being a nurse. As Sarah Trusselle, a Professional Development Nurse with experience of interviewing prospective nursing students and post-registration nurses, points out:

> There are fewer health sector jobs and more applicants. Competition is increasing.

The job description for a nurse has changed dramatically in the history of the role as was outlined in Chapter 1, and we are confident it will continue to evolve. Therefore anyone coming into nursing now needs to be confident of their skills and able to adapt within a workplace.

What are employability skills?

As well as your clinical skills and knowledge you need to be aware of the other skill sets you possess. These are sometimes known as 'employability skills'. Which skills these are will depend on who you are asking, but employers often have very definite ideas! Every year there will be two or three large-scale pieces of research with employers, investigating the skills gaps and their requirements from graduates from all subject areas.

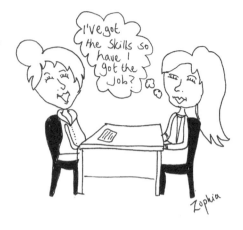

The variety of experiences, both positive and negative, that a nursing student has during the course of their training means that they will have evidence of using many skills, but often we fail to recognise and value the skills we are gaining.

The Confederation of British Industry (CBI) in its *Working Towards Your Future* report (CBI 2011) has worked with its members to define what employers mean by 'employability skills'. There are typical nursing experiences that might fit each skill:

- **Business and customer awareness** – basic understanding of the key drivers for business success, including the importance of innovation and taking calculated risks, and the need to provide customer satisfaction and build customer loyalty. Risk taking can be a part of a nurse's responsibility when it comes to prioritising tasks and care that needs to be delivered. In terms of customer satisfaction a nurse needs to be aware of quality in every aspect of delivery, of the patient experience and also that of the patient's carers and loved ones; as well as managing resources as effectively and efficiently as possible.
- **Problem solving** – analysing facts and situations and applying creative thinking to develop appropriate solutions. Problem solving for a nurse could be managing a breathless and confused patient; dealing with the emotions of carers; organising the ward area when staffing levels are low.
- **Communication and literacy** – application of literacy, ability to produce clear, structured written work and oral literacy, including listening and questioning. For a nurse, giving clear explanations, active listening and accurate recording are all integral to care planning and care delivery.
- **Application of numeracy** – manipulation of numbers, general mathematical awareness and its application in practical contexts (e.g. measuring, weighing, estimating and applying formulae). Calculation and administration of medication in appropriate amounts and at the appropriate time intervals are a major role of a nurse, as well as monitoring and interpreting patients' vital signs.
- **Application of information technology** – basic IT skills, including familiarity with word processing, spreadsheets, file management and use of internet search engines. Using different sorts of software for recording information, and technical expertise with equipment, are increasingly important in all nursing work.
- **A positive attitude** – underpinning all these attributes, the key foundation must be a positive attitude: a 'can-do' approach, a readiness to take part and contribute, openness to new ideas and a drive to make these happen. Given the rapidity of change within the nursing role and the technologies and techniques a nurse will use, an ability to cope with change – and be proactive in approach to it – is essential in a nurse. Alongside this is a willingness to keep up-to-date and be able to deliver evidence-based care.

- **Entrepreneurship/enterprise** (frequently mentioned by both employers and universities) – broadly, an ability to demonstrate an innovative approach, creativity, collaboration and risk taking. Multi-disciplinary team working in NHS contexts and collaboration with other agencies is imperative in nursing, as well as adopting creative approaches to patient recovery and welfare.

Because the language used by the CBI and other professions and employers is very 'business speak' many nursing students would not recognise their own qualities in that list. Language in recruitment is *very* important; it is all about understanding what employers are asking for and providing examples in a language the employer can understand. 'Translation' and 'transferability' are key to successful articulation of how perfectly you match the employer's requirements – translation of their 'recruitment speak', so that you can find the most relevant evidence in your portfolio of skills and experiences, and then write and speak about them in a language the recruiter understands; and transferability in terms of your understanding that your experiences in one context can easily also apply in a completely different context.

It is not easy to identify and articulate our skills and experiences and it does not come naturally to many of us. We are often uncomfortable talking about ourselves in a very positive way and don't like to 'big ourselves up'. However this skill of articulation and using appropriate language for the reader is vital for successful job hunting. There is more on this below.

Employability skills are not just gained from work experience – be that placement or paid employment – they are accumulated across our whole life. Some employers refer to 'well rounded' candidates, and by this they often mean people who bring an awareness of their life-wide experiences and skills. Elizabeth Bennett-Hayes who is a Senior Sister in Intensive Care and interviews for newly qualified nurse positions said:

> One candidate had said how she ran a Brownie group, which we liked due to the evidence of managing situations, responsibility and leadership. That particular application stuck in my mind.

The TargetJobs 'What employers want from graduate nurses' web page includes quotes from healthcare recruiters on the skills they are seeking – for example, interpersonal skills:

> Nursing is a unique skill. It requires a good knowledge base acquired through study, a nurturing, caring attitude, compassion, common sense, exceptional communication skills, and a grounded understanding of the social aspects of human responses and behaviours.
>
> Professor Irene Scott, Director of Nursing, Surrey and
> Sussex Healthcare NHS Trust

As we said earlier, employability is about valuing and recognising all of your experiences and how they are relevant for your career: organising that holiday for you and a number of friends; managing your own budget; responsibilities for dependants – siblings, children, parents, and so on; commitment to your own fitness and well-being – for example, regular attendance at a gym, dance class or football team.

Think about what you do in your spare time. Think of all the skills that are implicit in them. Let's take one – attending Zumba class once a week, for example. This involves being able to organise yourself, the ability to plan, demonstrate reliability and commitment whilst managing stressful situations with congruence, by which we mean that for a career in health you are also 'walking the walk' and an exemplar for future patients. Let's take another example – responsibility for ageing parents/grandparents. The skills implicit in this might include integrity and honesty, listening, problem solving, advocacy, organising and planning, reliability, compassion and empathy (for them and for yourself!).

One of the keys to employability is understanding how experiences in one area can be applied to another. We will go on to discuss this in more detail below, as this is crucial to convincing recruiters that you have what they want in abundance, so it is important that you not only recognise the value of all your experiences but record and review them! This will help you when it comes to completing application forms, in annual appraisal processes, completing your professional portfolio and making decisions about managing your career. If you have completed a skills audit or looked at a person specification and there are gaps, you can do something about it. If, in the recording of experiences process, you recognise how much you enjoyed or disliked an experience or skill, you might want to explore that further. The review process can help you make career decisions and choices – for example, identifying a specialism you want to pursue, a ward culture you really valued, a way of working you enjoy (perhaps one-to-one care or group care). It can also give you the confidence to seize opportunities and articulate your 'wonderfulness' or uniqueness in an interview or appraisal. It is important to recognise where you can add value, know how to sell yourself and stand out from the crowd of applicants. A record of your experiences might be in a paper or electronic portfolio – the vehicle is not important, the recording of the content is! (Casey and Egan 2010). These records are the basis for your CV or application form, *and* the stories you can tell with conviction in answer to an interview question like 'Give me an example of a time when you had to think on your feet'. How great would it be to have a lot of examples to choose from? (There is more on interviews below.)

Transferability

In the 40 plus years of our working lives we are likely to change jobs many times, and many of us will change careers a few times, so we need to be able to transfer learning from one job – one sphere of our lives – to another. Sometimes we will make the decision to change for ourselves, sometimes it will be forced upon us by circumstances beyond our control – for example, redundancy, our partner getting a job somewhere else in the country (or even in a different country), or other responsibilities making us want to change our working pattern and hours.

'Transferability' is a very good thing if we can articulate it as a strength and present it to ourselves and our potential employers as a desirable asset. Transferability (Thomas 2014) is also about being open to possibilities and seeing things from a different perspective. For example a nurse who says 'I only like working with medical patients' could increase their opportunities for work when they realise that district nursing is applying the same skills in a different setting.

Once you have trained as a registered nurse the opportunities for nursing are many and varied – for example, cruise ships, non-governmental organisations (NGOs), the pharmaceutical industry, medical supply companies, relevant professional organisations,

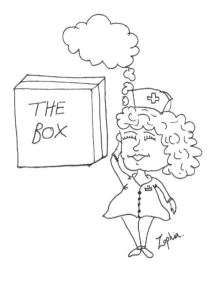

large public places like shopping centres and performance venues. Chapter 17, 'Nursing around the globe', provides you with a great insight into what to expect and will get you to think about your transferable skills. Thinking about your transferable skills should get you thinking outside of the box.

Transferability also means that you can take the skills and experiences of being a nurse and apply them to a completely different career – for example, teaching, publishing, armed services (Thomas 2014) and management of many kinds. In these circumstances it is vitally important that you understand how to *articulate* the value of the experience so that the 'new' career values it as much as you. For example, you will translate a 'nursing' experience into a 'hotel management' experience by converting . . .

I managed a 12-bed intensive care unit with over 100 staff. I had overall responsibility for recruitment and management of nursing staff, health and safety, risk assessment, hygiene, ordering of supplies, budget of £xmillion, training, education and ongoing professional development of staff, off-duty rotas, staff appraisal, policy writing and policy delivery, overseeing management and delivery of care, discharge and disaster planning.

. . . into something appropriate for hotel management, such as:

An experienced manager of a large disparate environment with many staff. Responsibility for day-to-day quality management and operational activities of over 100 staff including shifts and rotas. Responsibility for budget of £xmillion.

These skills of articulation and transferability will stand you in good stead in the next chapter, when we talk about applying for jobs as a nurse.

Summary

The key to employability is to be able to articulate and translate your experiences and skills into a language that is appropriate for the 'eye of the beholder'. When asked to rate employability skills compared to the specific occupational, technical or academic knowledge and skills associated with their degree, 82 per cent of graduate employers placed more importance on employability skills (CBI/EDI 2011).

References

Casey, D. and Egan, D. (2010) The use of professional portfolios and profiles for career enhancement. *British Journal of Community Nursing* 15(11): 547–552.

Confederation of British Industry and Education Development International plc. (2011) *Building for Growth: Business Priorities for Education and Skills: Education and Skills Survey 2011*. London: Confederation of British Industry, www.cbi.org.uk/media/1051530/cbi__edi_education___skills_survey_2011.pdf (accessed 18 March 2014).

Confederation of British Industry (2011) *Working Towards Your Future: Making the Most of Your Time in Higher Education*. London: Confederation of British Industry, http://educationandskills.cbi.org.uk/reports/00363 (accessed 18 March 2014).

TargetJobs 'What employers want from graduate nurses': http://targetjobs.co.uk/career-sectors/nursing-and-allied-healthcare-professions/applications-and-interviews/what-employers (accessed 18 March 2014).

Thomas, S. (2014) A force to be reckoned with. *Nursing Standard* 28(19): 64–65.

Further reading

Confederation of British Industry (2011) Universities and employability skills, www.cbi.org.uk/media-centre/press-releases/2011/05/universities-must-embed-employability-skills-in-course-structures-cbi-nus

Useful web links

Career planning/transferable skills: http://careerplanning.about.com/od/careerchoicechan/a/trans_skills_ex.htm

NHS Nursing careers: www.nhscareers.nhs.uk/explore-by-career/nursing

Royal College of Nursing/find a job in healthcare: www.rcn.org.uk/nursing/work_in_health_care/finding_a_job

Students diary/transferable skills: http://blogit.jamk.fi/studentsdiary/tag/transferable-skills.

Chapter 16

Securing your first job as a nurse

Ruth Lawton

This chapter will help you prepare to get started on your professional life as a nurse. We will look in detail at the eight rules for managing your career. These will ensure that you know what you have to offer, and where to look for opportunities, and that you succeed at interview and enjoy your working life.

The key to making – and keeping – ourselves employable is recognising and valuing our skills and experiences. We must record them so that we don't forget them and know how to present them – to ourselves to keep our confidence up, and to employers to prove we can do their job. I often talk to students about the 'eight rules for getting the best jobs for you' (see Box 16.1).

Think back to Chapter 9 when you were applying for the nursing programme. You had to prove that you had all of the skills, qualities, behaviours and attitudes appropriate for training as a nurse. The same thing applies to securing your first job as a nurse. Let's take each of the rules below and look at them in more detail.

Knowing the eight rules

Rule 1: Start early

It is important that you start to think about this really early in your nurse training because there are opportunities to learn about what you want from your career all the way through your study time.

Box 16.1 Eight rules for getting the best jobs for you

1   Start early.
2   Have all your evidence of your 'wonderfulness' to hand.
3   Make contacts and let them know you are keen and interested.
4   Do your research, not just into yourself but also into the job/organisation (Trust), sector, current issues in the profession and research.
5   Always match the person specification – that is what they want, prove you have it. Never lie!
6   At interview make sure you match how you presented yourself on paper – which of course means you are confident, passionate, honest, committed, smart, etc.
7   Get feedback.
8   Keep an eye on where you are and where you are going, and manage your own career.

Think about all of the placements you will do – each has something to teach you about a clinical speciality, cultures and management styles. You will also learn about yourself – what do you like and respond well to? As we said previously, it is important that you recognise and record (Casey and Egan 2010) all of these things so that you are ready to seize an opportunity when it presents itself – for example, knowing the timings for the nursing job market, keeping in touch with ward managers who you want to work for in the future, gathering the information you need to make the best decision for you.

Questions you could be asking yourself might include:

- Where are jobs advertised?
- Where do you want to work?
- How far are you prepared to travel (bearing in mind public transport and working shifts)?

To find out the answers you need to ask the right people.

If you start this process at the end of your studies it can take some time – during which you might miss the perfect job for you. Instead, work consistently on managing your career throughout your training so that you can continue in that good habit afterwards. This will bear you rich rewards and enable you to have more control over where you work, who you work with and what you are doing.

Job satisfaction is the reason for spending time thinking about you, and what you want. Which would you prefer – a job that didn't excite you or give you a feeling of fulfilment, with people you didn't really like, and in an environment that made you uncomfortable; or going to work with a spring in your step, with people who cared about you and who you cared about, and could have a laugh with, in a place that made you feel proud and purposeful?

Rule 2: Having evidence of your 'wonderfulness'

It is very hard for many of us to sing our own praises. We find it difficult to write – let alone say – nice things about ourselves. There is often a little voice that pops up in our head with ready examples to disprove whatever compliments we want to give ourselves.

You will have to learn to overcome this reluctance to present yourself in a positive, confident manner (and we will go into that below) but one easy way to help yourself is to keep a record of compliments. Look at the positive statements in the cartoon to the right. How much easier will it be to write 'My first placement report complimented me on my punctuality and reliability' or 'Amongst my circle of friends I am known as a good listener'.

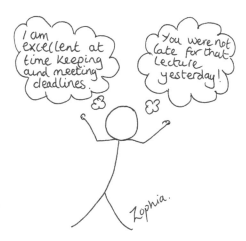

This record of compliments will be a part of the record you should keep of all your achievements, qualifications, skills, experiences and good qualities. People keep this information in many ways – from scraps of paper in a shoebox under the bed to an ePortfolio, with many digital layers of information.

We suggest you keep a 'DUMP CV'. DUMP stands for 'don't underestimate my potential', and this is where you can dump all of the evidence of your wonderfulness.

The DUMP CV is not the one you send to an employer. It is your total record of everything that makes you employable, so that when you do see the perfect job you can adapt and edit this CV to match the requirements the employer seeks. If you keep this on your computer and keep it up to date, when the perfect job comes around you will have everything you need to 'save as' and edit this into the perfect CV for that job, or 'copy and paste' all the best bits onto the application form. There is more about that below, when we look at Rules 4 and 5.

Rule 3: Make contacts and let them know you are keen and interested

By the time you graduate with your nursing degree you will have been on a number of placements – so you have the experience that employers seek. This is good news, as vacancies are expected to be filled by applicants who have already worked for the organisation during their studies (High Fliers Research 2013).

The world is small. Networks stretch across it easily. You have a good contacts list from your placements and they have their contacts, and if you ask one person for help you are potentially asking all the people they know too.

This means that it is important to try to maintain a good relationship with people you meet and work with on placement – even if there were aspects of the experience you did not like. These contacts may be:

- able to help you find opportunities elsewhere;
- a very useful, relevant referee on your application form or CV (see Rule 5 for why this is so important);
- your future employer or the person who puts you in touch with your future employer.

Networking is not about 'using people'. It is a two-way process, including being prepared to help others too, whether you are a student nurse or qualified nurse. In the twenty-first century it is not who you know that counts, but who knows you. Keep them sweet on you!

Using your network of contacts

There are two things you need to do to make sure that if any opportunities come up you are on hand and have a support system in place to hear about them:

1   Tell the people who do the recruiting that you want to work there – let them know you are interested.
2   Find out where they advertise their jobs, and make sure you check regularly.

Rule 4: Do your research

Do your research not just into yourself as outlined above but also into the job/organisation (Trust), sector, current issues. A personal visit can make a big difference. Sarah Trusselle, a

Professional Development Nurse with experience of interviewing prospective nursing students and post-registration nurses, says:

> Make the effort to go and look at the ward area or clinical environment where you will be possibly working – and ask questions such as what support you would be given, and find out what the job actually entails. Sometimes at interview the candidate has no awareness of what they have to do.

In addition, Katie Holmes, a careers consultant working with health professionals. says:

> Many Trust vacancies offer an orientation visit, but this is rarely taken up, so candidates who do take up such an offer are demonstrating initiative, enthusiasm and commitment.

Question: Where else will you find this information?
Answer: By using your network.

Where will you look for jobs?

Look where the jobs are advertised. Not just the formal places – for example:

- *Nursing Times:* www.nursingtimesjobs.com
- *Nursing Standard:* http://nursingstandard.rcnpublishing.co.uk
- Royal College of Nursing: www.rcnbulletinjobs.co.uk
- NHS website: www.jobs.nhs.uk
- Job centre and recruitment agencies (including specialist agencies) – see the Nursing Agencies list: www.nursing-agencies-list.com

... but also the informal places – for example, word-of-mouth, noticeboards in hospitals and the people in your network!

You see a job advertised that sparks your interest. You send for the information pack and back comes – via email – a job description and person specification and a link to an online application form. Most job descriptions will follow a similar format, with headings like:

1 Job Purpose – a summary of the role
2 Key Results – some targets for the role
3 Critical Activities – this might include professional activities and specialist skills, important transferable skills, education and training.

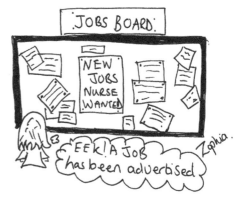

Rule 5: Always match the person specification

That is what they want, prove you have it. Never lie! A person specification is used by the employer to identify the 'essential' criteria for the role and also the 'desirable' criteria. If all candidates meet the essential requirements then the employer can include the desirable requirements to reduce and refine the shortlist. If you do not meet all of the 'essential' requirements it is unlikely that you will be shortlisted so you *must* write about these elements on your CV or application form. If you have the desirable requirements, then include them too, so that if there are lot of good candidates you can prove you are even better!

The person specification can help you to predict the sort of questions that will come up at the interview or the activities they may ask you to perform as part of the selection process. Graham Gordon – a Senior Nurse in Liver Services (retired) – stated that:

> The interview panel will agree a set of questions prior to the interview, based on the person spec, and we can't really deviate from that so it's crucial that you have examples that you can share and discuss.

Your next job is to prove that you have and can meet all of those requirements. This is where your up-to-date DUMP CV and portfolio will save you lots of time. You have all of the evidence of your wonderfulness, so all you have to do is choose the most appropriate and relevant examples. Sarah Trusselle, Professional Development Nurse, says:

> It is very important that you explain gaps – and think about who you use as a referee. The best reference is from someone who has line managed you in a clinical situation – including placement supervisors or a clinical assessor if you are about to qualify. For NHS posts, at least two referees are required and often an academic one as well.

Rule 6: At interview make sure you match how you presented yourself on paper

This, of course, means you are confident, passionate, honest, committed, smart, etc. We talked earlier about needing to write confidently about yourself. In an interview you need to be confident in person.

This doesn't mean you won't be nervous – your hands and voice might tremble, you might break out into a sweat or feel a cheesy grin stuck to your face – but these nerves are a sign of how much you want this job! Interviewers are usually nervous too – that's a sign of how important it is to them too.

But despite your nerves you will need to show the interviewer, or interview panel, that you meet all of their requirements. You already know what those requirements are because you have seen the person specification (Rule 5) and already proved in writing how wonderful you are.

Look back at Chapter 9 where we talked about preparing for interviews for nursing courses. Snow (2012) and Elcock (2012) also offer some really useful tips. That preparation and advice will be very useful when you are applying for your first nursing job. Here are some quick tips for interviews:

- Look at the person specification. What questions would you ask if you were the interviewer? Would you 'test' some of the competencies by asking candidates to demonstrate some skills? How would you test them? Now you know the sort of things you need to plan for/rehearse/anticipate.

- Are there any questions you want to ask the interview panel? If the answers are obvious don't ask them. Don't feel like you must have questions. A good selection process might include a 'briefing' where all your questions are answered.
- Show respect for the interviewers by looking smart and tidy and arriving on time (or a few minutes early).
- Be polite and interested with everyone you meet, including the other candidates, the receptionist, etc. Imagine that you are being watched from the moment you walk through the main doors, and behave accordingly.
- Remember that it is normal to be nervous, so try and help yourself by sitting up straight with your head up and shoulders back – this will help you to breathe better and also helps you to look and feel confident.
- Make eye contact with everyone on the panel but in particular with the person who asked you the question.
- It is OK to smile.
- Sometimes when we are nervous our 'mind goes blank' and you catch yourself rambling on and on, having forgotten the original question. Stop rambling. Ask them to repeat the question.

Sarah Trusselle told us that it was important that candidates don't overlook the obvious when thinking about how to answer interview questions:

> Make sure you talk about the basic fundamentals of patient care, not just the politics of NHS funding or professional issues.

Below are some general interview questions to help you practise talking about yourself in a positive, articulate way. Remember that the recruiter is looking for the candidate that matches their person specification and the best way you can do that is to give some examples of things you have done. By the time you have finished your nurse training you will have no trouble answering these questions I promise!

Katie Holmes has given us some examples of interview questions (Box 16.2) finding out about you, your skills, your nursing knowledge and your problem solving skills.

Box 16.2 Sample interview questions

- Why have you applied to us?
- Why should we offer you this position?
- Tell me about yourself
- What is your greatest strength or weakness?
- What would you contribute to this role?
- What practical and theoretical knowledge have you gained from your course?
- What did you find most difficult on your course?
- What would you say are your greatest skills?
- Can you give an example of a time when you have had to use your communication/analytical/problem solving skills in a work context?

These are general, so be prepared to be asked specialist and technical nursing field-specific questions.

The interview panel may also want to identify what you understand about professional development, so they may ask you questions such as:

- What do you understand by 'preceptorship'?
- What do you think your training needs will be?
- What does 'supervision' mean to you?
- What are your long-term goals?

Rule 7: Get feedback

It is imperative to know your strengths and areas for development in the recruitment process. So when the application/interview process is over, ask for feedback:

- if you are unsuccessful at any stage
- even when you are successful.

You can also give yourself some feedback by reflecting as soon as you can after an interview. Think about what went well or not so well, and compare your perception of how you did with feedback from the recruiter.

You can use your interview experiences to build up a store of typical questions to help you develop your technique and effectiveness at articulating your 'wonderfulness'. We talked earlier about networking being a two-way process – and this kind of interview experience is also something you can share with others.

Rule 8: Keep an eye on where you are and where you are going

This way, you manage your own career. Employability and career management are not just about getting your first job – that is simply employment. To manage your career you will undertake regular formal and informal reviews where you might ask yourself questions, such as:

- How am I doing with this job?
- Am I enjoying my work?
- Am I achieving all that I could?
- Am I up to date professionally?
- Is there anything I want to change?

Once you are qualified and in practice you will be required to think about your professional practice. No one will expect you to stay in the same job you started your career in, so you will need to keep an eye on your employability and career management skills, and make sure you can continue to articulate your wonderfulness!

When it comes to employability and nursing you can transfer everything you learn in your nursing training and experience to many other sectors and careers. All of the eight rules discussed earlier still apply for managing your career – whatever, whenever and wherever it is.

Summary

In this section we have looked at the rules you can follow to not only get your first job as a nurse but manage your career for many years afterwards – whether that be as a nurse or one of the many other opportunities for which you will be well equipped. As we outlined in Chapter 15, Employability – there are so many things a nurse can do, including working all over the world. If you take the approach that you will be learning all your life – new experiences, keeping up to date, maintaining your professional development – there are so many possibilities you can explore to keep you happy.

References

Casey, D. and Egan, D. (2010) The use of professional portfolios and profiles for career enhancement. *British Journal of Community Nursing* 15(11): 547–552.

Elcock, K. (2012) *Getting into Nursing.* London: Sage.

High Fliers Research (2013) *The Graduate Market in 2013: Annual Review of Graduate Vacancies and Starting Salaries at Britain's Leading Employers.* London: High Fliers Research, www.highfliers.co.uk/download/GMReport13.pdf (accessed 18 March 2014).

Snow, S. (2012) *Get into Nursing and Midwifery: A Guide to Application and Career Success.* Harlow: Pearson.

TargetJobs What employers want from graduate nurses, http://targetjobs.co.uk/career-sectors/nursing-and-allied-healthcare-professions/applications-and-interviews/what-employers (accessed 18 March 2014).

Further reading

Burke, L,. Sayer, J., Morris-Thompson, T. and Marks-Maran, D. (2014) Recruiting competent newly qualified nurses in the London region: An exploratory study. *Nurse Education Today*, www.nurseeducationtoday.com/article/S0260-6917(14)00040-9/abstract (accessed 18 March 2014).

Royal College of Nursing (2011) *RCN Career Service: Tips for Completing Application Forms and CVs.* London: Royal College of Nursing.

Useful web links

Job Seekers Guide: www.jobseekersguide.org

Mahara (example of an ePortfolio platform): https://mahara.org

PebblePad (example of an ePortfolio platform): www.pebblelearning.co.uk

Royal College of Nursing (CV clinic for nurses): https://shop.rcnpublishing.co.uk/ProductDetails.asp?ProductCode=CVCLINIC.

Chapter 17

Nursing around the globe

Debbie Pittaway, with Fang Yu and Anthony Tuckett

The opportunity to travel once qualified was perhaps one of the reasons that you chose a career in nursing in the first place. Or perhaps the desire to travel and work along the way has become an ambition. Or maybe you just want a change. Well, whatever your reason, you could not have chosen a career more mobile and more suited to travel and offering countless opportunities around the world.

My own experiences of travelling, and more importantly, actually working abroad, have given me some of the most memorable personal experiences, and enriched my professional life in so many ways. For me, this has been an amazing journey; but for the profession the need to develop an insight into global health issues and develop sound cultural awareness and sensitivity is a priority (Hancock 2008). Many of you may have had experience of this in your undergraduate education programme, either through Erasmus exchange or other curriculum content focusing on world health needs. Such an insight and experience will have undoubtedly helped to make you more aware of how geography, the global economy and natural phenomena impact on nursing care around the world in ways we could once only imagine.

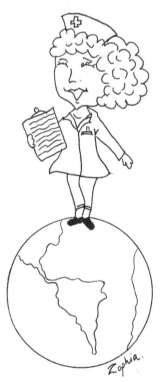

There is a whole world out there!

The world we live in is becoming smaller, and whilst travel costs are rising, the information technology revolution has made the world a more accessible place, both virtually and in reality. Such information affords you the opportunity to make informed choices about where and when you would like to work, and it gives you the chance to ask many of the questions that will make it possible and to then make that transition more smoothly. If you are travelling with family and perhaps children this type of knowledge will be crucial. Remember – despite the promises of tax-free earning and images of sandy beaches and never-ending sunshine, the reality of actually working and living abroad can be very different. You need to do your homework.

Being a nurse has enabled me to work in the most amazing places – from the chilly climes of Canada, to the

Far East, to Australia and the highlands of Papua New Guinea. I would never have imagined all of this when I started out at 18, but it is all possible. My colleagues, Fang and Anthony, who have contributed to this chapter, are just two of the people I have met along my way, and between us we hope to provide you with the detail that will help you make some of the choices which are so important when seeking to work around the world as a registered nurse. The chapter can only hope to give you an insight to some of the world – it is a big place – but if you gain anything, it will be a sense of how diverse it really is and how important it is to do the essential groundwork before embarking on your travels, wherever you choose to work.

Nursing elsewhere in the European Union

Europe covers a massive 10 million km^2 and comprises 49 countries, 28 of which form the European Union. Whilst a small continent by comparison to the Americas, for example, it is a diverse land mass – home to diverse populations, speaking a multitude of languages and bound by similarly diverse health and political systems. This diversity adds to the challenges of working in Europe, the biggest perhaps being the diversity of languages. When English is your first and only language the move to another country where the language is different presents a massive hurdle from the outset. If you are not prepared to learn a new language you will of course be narrowing your choices and reducing your options for employment. Obviously Ireland remains a possibility, or maybe some of the private clinics dotted around Europe, but your choice will certainly be narrowed. It is also worth noting that whilst we are able to travel freely on cheap flights around Europe without visas, the ability to practise as a registered nurse is more complex than simply jumping online and choosing your flight and grabbing your phrase book.

The intention of the Treaty of Rome (1957) is to enable members of the European Union to travel and work freely. However, it did not make the recognition of professional qualifications an obligation, making migrant movement, particularly of nurses, challenging.

Challenges have arisen as a consequence of the differing school systems up to the age of 18 years. This is then further compounded by a multiplicity of higher and further education systems. The Bologna Declaration (European Ministers of Education 1999) set in motion measures to address these issues, making it simpler to gain recognition for both your schooling and nurse education through a variety of processes. At its centre is the notion of 'mobility' and making it simpler for EU members to work within the Union. You should make the first port of call towards working within the EU the European Network of Information Centres (ENIC) and the National Academic Recognition Information Centres (NARIC). Both of these will assist you in determining the level of recognition of your school and professional education and qualifications. Very useful information can be found at www.enic-naric.net. It is important to understand that recognition of your qualifications is the first step in gaining employment within the rest of the EU as a registered nurse. Once you have done this, the process of securing work and the necessary registration requirements for the country of choice can begin.

Registration and regulation

The Nursing and Midwifery Council (NMC, www.nmc-uk.org) offer all registrants of the UK a comprehensive list of registering bodies outside the UK and of course the other EU countries are included. Here you will be able to access detailed information on how to gain registration in another member state and indeed advice regarding registration in any other country. It is a helpful second stop.

Given the number of countries in the EU, a detailed discussion about each is impossible, but a visit to the NMC website will quickly identify the appropriate authority to contact in the country of your choice. The European Council for Nursing Regulators (FEPI, www.fepi. org) offers other useful detail regarding regulation.

Visa information

You do not require a visa to work in another EU member state. However, remember that Europe is more than the EU, and as such you should always check visa or work permit requirements. A good place to start such enquiries is the Foreign and Commonwealth Office website (www.fco.gov.uk). Here you will find important contact details for all countries and, importantly, a list of British Embassies.

Finding a job

Finding a job may be your biggest hurdle. The issue of language means that other EU countries rarely advertise in the nursing press here in the UK. Most countries require a command of their official language. Coupled to the economic downturn of the last few years there has been a fall in job opportunities for English-speaking nurses in the EU. Finding a job in the EU may not be easy, but enquiries made to registering authorities within the country of choice may help you with useful employment leads. The obvious starting point for your search should be the myriad of employment agencies. Check the agencies' credentials, and perhaps seek recommendations. It is far better to have a positive experience – you will need lots of support, and clearly have many questions to ask. So you need to trust those offering advice and assistance.

Top tips

Language lessons

Plan well ahead. Maybe it is stating the obvious, but organising language lessons, registration and then employment all takes time. Staying on after an idyllic fortnight in the sun hoping to find employment is perhaps a little naive. But doing your homework and planning for such a move may well make your dreams possible. A first visit to the BBC (www.bbc.co.uk/languages) may help you start this process with some valuable early language tips.

This is a free service but really helps with testing your skills. After you have dipped your toe in here it is advisable to contact local colleges and language schools to get you off to the best possible start in your new country.

Finances

Financial considerations are so important, and whilst a move elsewhere in Europe may not involve the expense of relocation to the other side of the world, there are costs involved, and you must consider how these will impact upon the choices that you are able to make.

You need to appreciate the impact the currency exchange will have upon any earnings and how taxation will be managed. So often the fact that you may be taxed on your worldwide income is not considered. It is therefore wise to seek financial advice on all taxation matters when you know you are moving. The last thing you need is a tax bill as a welcome home gift. A good place to start is Her Majesty's Revenue and Customs website (HMRC, www. hmrc.gov.uk/cnr). Here you can seek relevant details and advice regarding your personal tax situation.

Nursing in the United Arab Emirates

As with a move to any new country, perhaps the best way to begin is by gaining a 'lived experience' in the United Arab Emirates (UAE). A visit may be costly but it will pay dividends in the long run. Glossy brochures and exhibitions here at home cannot give you the sense of the country and what it really is like to live there. The region is an amazingly vibrant and busy place; modern architecture with the backdrop of blue seas on one side and the vastness of the desert on the other. The sights and sounds will take your breath away.

The opportunities for work as a nurse here are similarly diverse and plentiful. In 2010 it was estimated that the nursing workforce in the Emirates needed to increase by 30 per cent. This shortage continues, with vacancies across most specialties. The opportunities for those with at least two years' post-qualifying experience are clear. Vacancies can be found again at the plethora of nursing and employment agencies. Whilst the ability to speak Arabic is an added advantage this is not always a requirement for an appointment here. Many of the positions are in private clinics and hospitals, many of them American.

Registration and regulation

Your first point of contact should be the NMC. They offer an excellent starting point for advice for anyone contemplating a career outside Europe (www.nmc-uk.org/Registration/ Planning-to-work-outside-the-UK/Planning-to-work-outside-of-Europe). Here you will be able to start to understand how much you need to do before you embark on job searches and booking flights again!

The Royal College of Nursing (RCN) offer an excellent insight into what you need to do when seeking to work abroad (www.rcn.org.uk/nursing/workingabroad?SQ_ACTION= login&). You do need to be a member of the RCN to access this detail but if you are, it really is very valuable and can prevent you searching in multiple places for answers to some common questions. Their support can continue after your move, with indemnity insurance (except for the United States and Canada), which is so important with any relocation abroad.

The International Council of Nurses (www.icn.ch/about-icn/about-icn) provides information regarding working in many countries and is helpful to understand the political, social and economic context of the country.

The Emirates Nursing Association (www.ena.ae) provides you with an insight into the work of the nurse in the UAE, the history of the role, and the passion that they have for developing, raising the profile and strengthening the professional role of the nurse in Emirate society.

Registering to practise as a nurse in the UAE needs to be organised through the Ministry of Health UAE, Federal Department of Nursing (www.nas.moh.gov.ae/RR.aspx). Here you can obtain advice regarding registering to work in any of the states. This link takes you directly to the detail required for verification and registration. If you gain an offer of employment your new employer will often help you to organise registration but it is much more impressive if you can start this process yourself!

Visa information

You will require a visa to work in the UAE. To obtain one you will need to have secured a confirmed offer of a job and sponsorship from an employer. Advice and guidance regarding visas can be obtained from the UAE Embassy (www.uaeembassyuk. net). Further details can be obtained from the Foreign and Commonwealth Office website (www.fco.gov.uk) about living and working outside the UK, and also about British Embassies overseas.

Finding a job

The nursing press here in the UK has for years been awash with opportunities for suitably qualified nurses in the Middle East. With the promise of endless sunshine and tax-free salaries the region has long been a draw for nurses.

Salaries are good and available accommodation excellent. Private medical insurance is included in salary packages – and essential if you are contemplating such a move. Flights back home once per year may also be included in a salary package and, in some cases, incentive packages for education if you are moving with children under the age of 18. But the cost of living has risen over the last few years, so as with all countries around the world you would be very wise to make calculations before taking the plunge. Tax-free earnings are a bonus, but you must ensure that you are fully compliant with your tax obligation in the UK before you leave and also your tax requirements whilst abroad. This obligation is bound by residency requirements. Guidance and advice should be sought before you leave the UK (www.hmrc.gov.uk/cnr). This way you'll have no nasty surprises should you return to the UK.

Top tips

It is vital to do your homework and don't underestimate the implication and cost of living of working abroad. If you can, I strongly advise you to invest in a fact-finding visit – live and breathe this amazing region before taking the plunge and relocating to do so. It is a big move and you are making a commitment to the health of the region.

Consider your lifestyle needs and wants. If popping to see your Mum once a week is a must – think on, this won't be possible! Unless that is you want a shed load of air miles!

Nursing in Australia

Australia is a big place. It covers nearly 8 million square kilometres – you could cookie-cutter 31 UKs from that! If you've got a relative in Melbourne (Victoria) and you get a job in Brisbane (Queensland) that's 1700 km or about a 20-hour car drive for a nice cup of tea! Australia is also a long way away from the UK – it will take you about 26 hours by plane to get there, so not too many quick trips home for a birthday or the European Cup Final.

Australians talk differently – the accent can be quite flat and broad, and some Aussies mumble whilst others end a conversation with 'Heh?' You will know that you are in a special place and your nursing career of a diamond standard when your newly admitted patient on the ward says: 'G'day mate! Where's the dunny?'

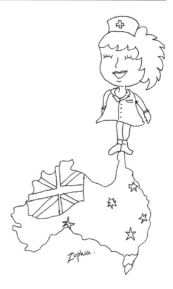

Well-meaning humour aside, you are advised to do some research about contemporary Australia and Australians before coming on down. The Australian Government Department of Immigration and Citizenship gives a fantastic flavour of what life is like 'down under', and you can get a real insight into what the country has to hold for you and your family (www.immi.gov.au/living-in-australia/choose-australia). It also provides a deeper understanding of the important ideals that make Australia what it is. You can really begin to understand the principles that the country has been built on.

The nursing workforce 'down under'

Most nurses in Australia work in acute care hospitals. Typically though, a reasonable number work in residential aged care facilities (nursing homes) and in the community (home-visiting and community health centres). As elsewhere, nursing skills and what nurses do varies depending on what type of care is required and on the care setting.

In 2009 there were some 280,000 nurses (including midwives) working in Australia, of whom 80 per cent were clinical nurses. Australian nurses are getting older, are still predominantly female, and two-thirds of them work in the public health system.

For more information on the Australian nursing and midwifery workforce, the Australian Institute of Health and Welfare (www.aihw.gov.au/nursing-midwifery-work-force), the Department of Health and Ageing (www.health.gov.au/internet/main/publishing.nsf/Content/work-nurse) and the Australian Nursing Federation (www.anf.org.au/pdf/Fact_Sheet_Snap_Shot_Nursing.pdf) provide excellent detail and insight into the role of the nurse.

Employers

In Australia nurses make up nearly half the total health workforce and are employed in the public sector – more than any of the other professions. Seventy percent of Australian nurses work in acute care hospitals, mental health services, residential aged care facilities (nursing homes), community health services (home-visiting and community health centres), hospices and schools (Department of Health and Ageing, 2012).

Australian nurses work in the major cities – Canberra, Melbourne, Sydney, Brisbane, Darwin, Perth and Adelaide – but opportunities also abound beyond the coastline in rural and remote areas. To find out about rural and remote areas of nursing, Queensland Health provide valuable detail regarding this unique and rewarding area of practice (www.health.qld.gov.au/nursing/rural_remote.asp).

Show me the money

While there is some degree of consistency, nurses and midwives' wages and conditions can vary depending on the relevant state (Queensland, Western Australia, South Australia, Victoria, New South Wales) or territory (Australian Capital Territory, Northern Territory) and the specific area of nursing. For a sense of wages in Queensland, see www.health.qld. gov.au/hrpolicies/wage_rates/nursing.asp, and for Western Australia, see www.nursing. health.wa.gov.au/docs/working/wages.pdf.

Registration and regulation

All nurses in Australia must be registered to practise with the Nursing and Midwifery Board of Australia (NMBA) which is responsible for regulating the profession. The application form (AGOS-40) for general registration (graduated or trained overseas nurse/midwife) is submitted through the Australian Health Practitioner Regulation Agency (AHPRA) (ANF, 2012; NurseInfo, 2012). Very useful information is available from the Australian Health Practitioner Regulation Agency (www.ahpra.gov.au) and the NMBA (www. nursingandmidwiferyboard.gov.au) where you can download an AGOS-40 application form. The site also provides some helpful supplementary information when you are completing the form. This will help prevent you making mistakes and will of course speed up the whole process for you.

Visa information

Excellent Visa information for international nurses and midwives is available at the Australian Nursing Federation website (www.anf.org.au). Here you will be able to locate your visa options and choices. This is particularly helpful if you are not using an agency to relocate.

Have your visa issued before applying for a job. Visa application can take some time and a potential employer is better served when you know your date of arrival and have secured a visa to work.

Finding a job

Check out some of the following websites:

- Nursing Careers Allied Health: www.ncah.com.au
- Nursing Jobs: www.nursingjobs.com.au
- Jobs 4 Nurses: www.jobs4nurses.com.au

Other useful sites

- www.health.vic.gov.au/nursing/becoming/overseas (Victorian Government health information for international nurse and midwife graduates);
- http://nursing.sesiahs.health.nsw.gov.au/Overeas_Qualified_Nurses_and_Midwives/ index.asp (New South Wales Health Department information for overseas qualified nurses and midwives);

- www.nursingsa.com/nursing_overseas.php (Nursing and Midwifery Office of South Australia, information for internationally educated nurses and midwives);
- Western Australia Health European Office phone: (+44) 020 7395 0575; email: health@wago.co.uk.

Top tips

English language skills

There are very specific language requirements and a number of countries including Canada, Republic of Ireland, South Africa, UK and the USA are recognised by the NMBA for the purpose of this regulatory standard. It is essential that you read the fact sheet and frequently asked question section (www.nursingmidwiferyboard.gov.au/Codes-Guidelines-Statements/FAQ.aspx).

Some of you will have to sit the International English Language Test System (IELTS) exam or the Occupational English Test (OET). Be sure to read what is required (see Questions 26–28 on the AGOS-40 form).

Apply before you depart

To save time, start the nurse registration process before arriving in Australia. The process can take 4–6 weeks (AHPRA 2012).

Recruitment agency

Think about using a recruitment agency specialising in placing international nursing and midwifery staff in Australia. Do your homework though – and ask about. Agents are not all the same and not usually cheap.

Nursing in the United States

Understanding nursing in the US

In 2011, nurses topped the Gallup poll for the 12th time as the most trustworthy professionals by the US public, in the 13 years that they had been included as an option. Nurses only lost their first spot in 2001 to firefighters in the wake of the September 11 terrorist attacks.

As one of the highest paid occupations, nursing faces a critical shortage in the coming decades. Domestic strategies to boost the nursing workforce are challenged by a shortage of faculty and clinical education sites which resulted in 52,115 qualified applicants being turned away in 2010. The gap created by nursing vacancies as a result of a reduced number of nurses being trained means that there are many opportunities for nurses trained in the UK to secure jobs working in the US.

Another strong appeal of US nursing is its career ladder for registered nurses (RNs): from baccalaureate to Master's to doctoral degrees (Doctor of Nursing Practice – DNP and Doctorate of Philosophy – PhD). The Master's and DNP prepare students as Advanced Practice Registered Nurses (APRNs) in four tracks: Certified Nurse Anaesthetist (CRNA),

Certified Nurse Midwife (CNM), Clinical Nurse Specialist (CNS), and Nurse Practitioner (NP). While the majority of PhD nurses work in academic settings, many conduct research clinically.

Several organisations, including the National League for Nursing (www.nln.org/careers/index.htm), the American Association of Colleges of Students (www.aacn.nche.edu/students) and others (e.g. www.allnursingschools.com), offer some helpful detail about nursing careers in the US.

The nursing workforce

Nursing is the largest healthcare profession in the US, with more than 3.1 million RNs. From 1980 to 2008, the educational levels of RNs have increased from 18% to 36% holding an associate's degree and from 22% to 37% having a bachelor degree, and decreased from 55% to 14% with a hospital diploma. About 13% of RNs had a master's or doctoral degree in 2008. The *Future of Nursing* report (Institute of Medicine 2010) called for 80% of the nursing workforce to hold at least a bachelor's degree by 2020.

The current unemployment rate for RNs is 1.1%. RN jobs are estimated to grow 26% from 2010 to 2020, making it one of the fastest growing occupations. The nursing shortage is projected to grow to 260,000 RNs by 2025.

The American Association of Colleges of Students (www.aacn.nche.edu/research-data) provides an essential insight and understanding of the American nursing workforce.

Employers

RNs are employed at a variety of settings. In May 2011, about 30% of RNs worked in general medical and surgical hospitals, 16% in outpatient centres, 14% in home care services, 10% in physician offices, 8% in long-term care facilities, and 22% in others.

You can learn about major employers by exploring the following organisations. The American Hospital Association (www.aha.org) within its member 'constituency sections' provides important detail regarding different employers. Similarly the American Association for Long Term Care Nursing (www.ltcnursing.org/healthcare-partners.htm) and the National Association for Home Care & Hospice (www.nahcagencylocator.com) will help you gain a sense of the types of employers in the US.

Salary opportunities

Average nurse salaries vary by educational levels, geographical locations, and practice settings, e.g.:

* Government: $68,540
* Hospitals; state, local, and private: $67,210
* Home health care services: $62,090
* Nursing and residential care facilities: $58,830
* Offices of physicians: $58,420

The average salaries for RNs and nursing faculty were $65,470 per year in 2012. Data from the Bureau of Labor Statistics (BLS) report that the lowest 10 per cent of registered nurses earned less than $45,040 and the top 10 per cent earned in excess of $94,720. The BLS website (www.bls.gov/oes/current/oes291111.htm) will give you a better sense of current RN wages.

Registration and regulation

Nurses must possess a licence from the state where they want to work. The initial RN licence is obtained by meeting the educational requirement and passing the Standardized National Council Licensure Examination (NCLEX)–RN through one of the fifty State Boards of Nursing. Having an RN licence in one state allows nurses to apply for RN licences in other states by endorsement.

To qualify for the NCLEX-RN exam, foreign nurses must hold an initial licence as a first-level, general nurse in their country of nursing education, demonstrate English proficiency (i.e. TOEFL), and have a verification of their nursing education and credentials by the Commission on Graduates of Foreign Nursing Schools (CGFNS International®). One of two CGFNS services is required for taking the NCLEX-RN exam: Credentials Evaluation Service, or CGFNS Qualifying Exam®. Once qualified, foreign nurses can take the NCLEX-RN exam in one of the fifty states, or one of the foreign NCLEX locations (UK (London), Germany, Hong Kong, South Korea (Seoul), Australia, India, Japan, Mexico, Canada, or Taiwan).

Very useful information is available at: www.allnursingschools.com/nursing-careers/career/nursing-state-boards (complete list of state boards of nursing); www.cgfns.org (CGFNS International®); www.ncsbn.org/2911.htm (National Council of State Boards of Nursing).

Visa information

Although employers will apply for a work visa or permanent residence for foreign nurses, it is a good idea to hire your own immigration attorney to help the process. RN licences might not be issued without social security numbers, but passing the NCLEX-RN exam or CGFNS Qualifying Exam®, and/or the CGFNS International® VisaScreen® is usually sufficient.

You can explore useful information about visas, immigration and citizenship at the US Citizenship and Immigration Services (www.uscis.gov/portal/site/uscis).

Further information to support this process and inform your application can be found at:

- www.cgfns.org/sections/programs/vs;
- www.usimmigrationsupport.org/h2b-work-visa.html (work visa for college educated professionals);
- www.usimmigrationsupport.org/h1b-work-visa.html (work visa for skilled and unskilled workers);
- The American Bar Association (www.americanbar.org) can help you locate a credentialled immigration attorney to help complete your application process.

Finding a job

The following web links are valuable sources of information when researching jobs in the US:

- www.nursingworld.org (American Nurses Association);
- www.nursingcenter.com (Lippincott's Nursing Center);
- www.monster.com (links to jobs around the globe);
- www.nurse.com (links to jobs across all states in different settings);
- www.nursepath.com (job search website).

Other useful sites

- www.bls.gov/ooh/Healthcare/Registered-nurses.htm#tab-6 (occupational outlook handbook for RNs).
- www.fiercehealthcare.com/story/house-passes-foreign-nurse-bill-serve-shortage-areas/2011-08-04 (House Passes Foreign Nurse Bill to Serve Shortage Areas).
- http://travel.state.gov/visa (US Department of State).

Top tips

Step 1 Identify a state where you want to apply for an RN licence by exam

- Complete all requirements from the State Board of Nursing:
  - Take the English proficiency test such as TOEFL (www.ets.org/toefl) if required;
  - Complete all CGFNS services required.
- Prepare, take, and pass the NCLEX-RN exam.

Step 2 Find a job

- Find a job in the state where you pass the NCLEX-RN exam or hold an RN licence;
- Have an employer sponsor your work or immigrant visa;
- Hire an immigration lawyer to help visa application.

Step 3 Move to the US

Move to the US after you have obtained your visa.

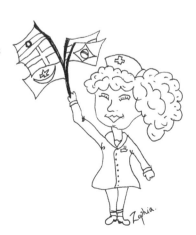

Summary

We have included a lot of detail here and only really skimmed the surface about working in four regions of the world. There are so many more places, but I think that what we have been able to convey is an idea of some of the crucial steps that will help you make a move to work as a nurse in another country more smoothly.

Of course there is so much more than just gaining a visa, your registration and a job. It is about experiencing new health systems, new people, and new cultures and sometimes giving up your old life, at least for a while. It can be very scary, particularly taking your whole family with you, but also so exciting. You will encounter so much out there that is impossible to imagine. And if you do choose to come home to the UK, those experiences will stay and enrich your personal and professional life in many ways for a long time into the future.

It sounds clichéd but it is so true – there honestly is a 'whole world out there' for you to explore, and I can't think of a better career to take you on that journey.

References

American Association of Colleges of Nursing (AACN) (2010) *Nursing schools forced to turn away thousands of qualified applicants.* http://nursing.advanceweb.com/News/National-News/50000-Qualified-Nursing-School-Applicants-Turned-Away-in-2010.aspx (accessed 20 February 2014).

Australian Health Practitioner Regulation Agency (AHPRA) (2012) *Registration Process: How long will my application take to process?* www.ahpra.gov.au/Registration/Registration-Process.aspx (accessed 3 March 2014).

Australian Nursing Federation (ANF) (2012) *Nursing in Australia: Overseas Nurses,* www.anf.org.au/html/about_nursing.html (accessed 2 March 2014).

Brush, B.L., Sochalski, J. and Berger, A.M. (2004) Imported care: Recruiting foreign nurses to U.S. health care facilities. *Health Affairs,* 23(3): 78–87.

Department of Health and Ageing (2012) *Nursing Workforce,* www.health.gov.au/internet/main/publishing.nsf/Content/work-res-ruraud-toc~work-res-ruraud-2~work-res-ruraud-2-3~work-res-ruraud-2-3-nurs (accessed 2 March 2014).

Emirates Nursing Association, www.ena.ae (accessed 5 January 2014).

European Ministers of Education (1999) The Bologna Declaration, www.ec.europa.eu/education/policies/educ/bologna/bologna.pdf (accessed 2 February 2014).

European Network of Information Centres and the National Academic Recognition Information Centres, www.enic-naric.net. (accessed 2 January 2014).

Foreign and Commonwealth Office, www.fco.gov.uk (accessed 2 January 2014).

Hancock, C. (2008) *The Globalisation of Nursing.* Oxford: Radcliffe Publishing.

Her Majesty's Revenue and Customs, www.hmrc.gov.uk/cnr (accessed 5 January 2014).

International Council for Nurses, www.icn.ch/about-icn/about-icn/ (accessed 5 March 2014).

Institute of Medicine (2010) *The Future of Nursing: Leading Changes, Advancing Health,* www.refworks.com/refworks2/default.aspx?r=references MainLayout::init (accessed 10 March 2014).

Jones, J.M. (2011) *Record 64% rate honesty, ethics of Members of Congress low: Ratings of nurses, pharmacists, and medical doctors most positive,* www.gallup.com/poll/151460/Record-Rate-Honesty-Ethics-Members-Congress-Low.aspx (accessed 2 April 2014).

Ministry of Health, United Arab Emirates, Federal Department of Nursing. www.nas.moh.gov.ae/RR.aspx (accessed 5 January 2014).

NurseInfo (2012) Nursing and midwifery in Australia: How to apply for registration, www.nurseinfo.com.au/overseas/registration (accessed 3 March 2014).

Nursing and Midwifery Council, www.nmc-uk.org (accessed 2 January 2014).

Nursing and Midwifery Council, www.nmc-uk.org/Registration/Planning-to-work-outside-the-UK/Planning-to-work-outside-of-Europe/ (accessed 5 January 2014).

Royal College of Nursing, www.rcn.org.uk/nursing/workingabroad?SQ_ACTION=login& (accessed 5 January 2014).

The Treaty of Rome (1957), www.ec.europa.eu/economy_finance/emu_history/documents/treaties/rometreaty2.pdf (accessed 2 January 2012).

United Arab Emirates Embassy United Kingdom, www.uaeembassyuk.net/ (accessed 5 January 2014).

Chapter 18

Embarking on a journey of lifelong learning

Tony Whittle and Cathy Poole

Long gone are the days when student nurses completed their nurse training and put their academic learning on hold to concentrate on development of their clinical skills. We are now in the era of 'lifelong learning'. The professional responsibility to keep up to date with new and innovative ways of working which are evidence-based forms the foundation of nurses' ability to declare themselves fit to remain on the professional nursing register. This professional responsibility is strongly linked to nurses' individual personal development and there is an expectation that all nurses will actively seek out new learning opportunities. This fosters the acquisition of new skills and serves as a driver for career development. Guy (2006) acknowledges that nurses' careers which were once planned by their employers are now seen very much as sitting in the employees' domain. Training is therefore no longer viewed as a one-off event but more as a learning journey which gathers and expands transferable skills. As a registered nurse you will enter a lifelong learning career path where you will be expected to mix your nursing skills with ongoing study – it's like being split in two.

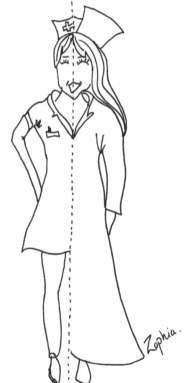

This approach to lifelong learning is aligned to what is commonly termed continuous professional development (CPD). That is, your personal development is one way to your own personal and professional success, and this development is not one-off, but is ongoing and lifelong, enabling you to gain skills and knowledge to further your personal and professional aims.

Once qualified it may be that the last thing on your mind is what next in terms of continuing your studies and how you begin to build on your initial registration by broadening and increasing your specialist knowledge and skills. Or it might be that you already have an idea of what you would like to do next and need to find out how you can achieve your aims in terms of qualifications and professional personal development. Wherever you might be, this chapter aims to help and provide you with some thoughts and ideas on how you can continue your professional development.

Continuous professional development

Continuous professional development can be 'credit bearing' or 'non-credit bearing'. Most of this chapter deals with credit-bearing CPD, but a lot of CPD can be non-credit bearing. Examples of this may be short 1-day, 2-day or 3-day courses in communication, palliative care, end-of-life care or 'preceptorship', for example. (Preceptorship is a defined programme which is designed to help newly qualified healthcare professionals to make the transition from student to qualified practitioner in a supportive environment.) These may be delivered in-house by organisations, or by private companies specialising in specific nursing and health areas. Non-credit-bearing CPD is an excellent way of updating knowledge and awareness of current issues for many nurses, with a certificate of attendance providing evidence and it has the advantage of no formal assessment!

Many departments/wards/units provide initial CPD in the form of preceptorship and role foundation. The focus of these can vary from dedicated course preceptorship for a group of nurses as they adapt to their new role, to a competence-based programme specifically in areas such as intensive care. Many units/departments have attached academic credits to their in-house induction/role-preparation programme through partnership working with local higher education institutions (HEIs) which enhances the value of the courses to the participant.

Why CPD?

CPD is important. It is important for you personally and professionally – which is why it is sometimes referred to as 'continuous personal and professional development' (CPPD).

It is also important for your organisation, and ultimately it is important for your patients so that they receive the highest quality evidence-based care, based on knowledge and skills acquired through your development.

CPD is becoming increasingly important for you – to enhance your role and the quality of the care you deliver now and how you meet the requirements of your current band/job description. But it is also important to consider what CPD is required to meet the requirements of the next band upwards in order for your career to progress. If you want to seek promotion then you must attain the fundamental qualifications required for that job.

CPD is, of course, a fundamental requisite to remain on the NMC register. The next section of this chapter outlines what the NMC (2011) expectations are in relation to registered nurses' ability to demonstrate their CPD through the 'Post-registration education and practice' standard, commonly referred to as Prep (NMC 2011). The requirement to be able to demonstrate CPD through Prep is an essential step which allows a registered nurse to re-register with the NMC and thus maintain their licence to practise as a nurse, as outlined in Chapter 10. This re-registration requirement is currently under review by the NMC. It is consulting key stakeholders under the term 'revalidation' which will ultimately change the requirements for nurses and midwives to maintain their registration. This revalidation process is being piloted in six sites (see pages 100–101) with the view that the new process will be in place by the end of 2015.

Currently, collating evidence of your ongoing CPD is really useful and it is recommended that this evidence is gathered in the form of a personal portfolio (Casey and Egan 2010) or profile of evidence. The Royal College of Nursing (2010) have embraced this concept and have developed an online resource through their learning zone which allows you to develop an electronic portfolio (ePortfolio) which you may find useful to take a look at. Portfolios and profiles are particularly useful when you are demonstrating your CPD as evidence to support your re-registration with the NMC (2011) and, importantly, can be used to support your application for new jobs.

The NMC (2011) Prep requirements

The Prep requirements are professional standards set by the NMC. They are legal requirements, which all registered nurses must achieve to enable their registration with the NMC to be renewed. Two separate Prep standards are identified which affect your ability to re-register.

The Prep (practice) Standard

You must have worked in some capacity by virtue of your nursing or midwifery qualification during the previous three years for a minimum of 450 hours, or have successfully undertaken an approved 'Return to Practice' course within the last three years (NMC 2011: 4).

The Prep (continuing professional development) Standard

You must have undertaken and recorded your continuing professional development over the three years prior to the renewal of your registration. All nurses and midwives have been required to comply with this standard since 1995. Since 2000, nurses have had to declare on their Notification of Practice (NoP) form that they have met this requirement when they renew their registration (NMC 2011: 4). This is in essence a self-declaration which is made confirming that the registrant has kept themselves up to date and can therefore renew their registration and continue to Practise as a registered nurse.

The NMC are currently undertaking a full review of the revalidation requirements and as a consequence of that review there will be some changes to the current Prep requirements which are set to come into force by December 2015.

A major CPD consideration has recently evolved. The reason for this is that during 2012 there was a move towards the all-graduate status of nursing. What this means is that if you apply to undertake pre-registration training today it will be at degree level, and in some instances at Master's level. In the past you could either train at certificate, diploma or degree level. Therefore it is important to carefully assess what level you have already studied at in order for you to undertake CPD to the next academic level. We call this 'academic progression'.

So what does this mean in reality? If you are a Diplomat Registered Nurse or a Certificate Registered Nurse, then for you the most important aspect of CPD may well be how you can become a graduate. If this is your primary aim, then how do you go about achieving your graduate status – a BSc (Hons), for example? You need to see what professional development opportunities there are available and start researching which ones suit your needs, as no one single approach suits all.

Location and types of CPD delivery

In pursuit of CPD you should consider what your local HEI (i.e. university) is and research what they provide in terms of credit-bearing courses at degree (level 6) or postgraduate

(7) level, or whether the courses on offer are non-credit-bearing. If you are looking to 'top up' your diploma to a degree, you need to establish if they offer awards to help you to achieve this. The Open University, which delivers courses via a distance learning approach, is a popular choice for some registered nurses. Distance learning/e-learning is becoming a more common feature of what is provided within CPD. However you need to consider if this mode of learning suits you.

Many providers of CPD offer what is often referred to as 'blended courses' which provide a mixture of taught content at the education institution and electronic-based materials which you can access remotely. Electronic access is particularly useful if you are trying to juggle work, study and family commitments – a situation which many learners pursuing CPD find themselves in. Additionally e-learning courses are especially advantageous if the CPD you want to undertake is some distance from where you live and can therefore save you time and, importantly, some travel costs.

What qualifications/academic credits do you already have?

This may seem a simple question to ask but, as with many simple questions, these can be the most valuable. Some thoughts and personal questions to consider are outlined in Box 18.1.

As discussed earlier, this is where an ePortfolio/profile or CV is vitally important as a record of your achievements to date. It can be considered as a collated record of your current achievements, evidence of learning and of the knowledge and skills you have gained as outlined in Chapter 16. Ideally it should also contain evidence of your reflection on practice, demonstrating links to clinical practice (NMC 2011; RCN 2010). Your ePortfolio/profile is therefore your way of collecting and maintaining records of your activities and learning events (which may be credit-bearing or non-credit-bearing) that demonstrates your ability to re-register – but also shows your employability with regard to jobs in the future. As Chapter 16 also pointed out, it can be a fantastic place to 'dump' all your evidence, as you never know when you may need to call upon the content and use it to help you make career choices and, of course, CPD choices.

So ideally if you are choosing to access a credit-bearing programme of study you need to plan it to suit your needs, and ensure that the study you undertake can be used as a stepping

---

Box 18.1 Questions to consider prior to CPD choice

- What have I already done in terms of CPD?
- Were any of the courses credit-bearing? The usual way of remembering is by asking yourself whether there was an assessment with this course.
- Was it linked to a university/college?
- What records or evidence do I have of the modules/units attended?
- Is this evidence in my ePortfolio/profile/CV?
- How many credits do I already have?
- Are these credits still current?
- When did I qualify?
- Was it at diploma level (level 5)?
- Was it at degree level (level 6)?

stone towards a degree, a postgraduate qualification (Postgraduate Certificate/Postgraduate Diploma or MSc award) or even to help you climb the career ladder and get that job you have been dreaming of.

APEL

APEL stands for 'accreditation of prior experiential learning'. It is a method whereby you are able to demonstrate that you have previous knowledge and skills attained through work or life experiences (Betts 2010). Universities operate their APEL in slightly different ways. However the end result of an individual university APEL process is that it allows you to evidence your previous experiences and therefore negates the need for you to repeat learning that you have already done. The APEL process will require you to provide robust evidence of your previous learning, so keeping a record (ePortfolio/profile/DUMP CV) becomes an increasingly important part of your CPD, because it recognises the lifelong learning you have achieved and how it can be maximised in terms of value through APEL. In general terms, therefore, APEL accepts the belief that all learning should be recognised.

What subject to study?

Nursing has historically based its post-registration framework on what I call 'kitemark' courses. These are courses that are seen as essential to gaining promotion and undertaking higher band roles within a specific area of nursing practice. Many years ago these kitemark courses were known as English National Board (ENB) courses. ENB courses in burns, coronary care or tissue viability, for example, were required in order for nurses to gain promotion and progress their careers. The descendants of these courses can still be seen in many Post-registration/Learning Beyond Registration courses provided within HEIs. So if you are considering working in a particular speciality it would be worthwhile identifying the relevant kitemark course and finding out how accessible it is for you. And does that speciality regularly send staff on these courses? You now need to ask yourself some more questions and, most importantly, do some research, for example:

- How would you gain a place?
- When is the course delivered?
- What are the time/study commitments?
- How are the courses financed?
- Who should I contact to find out?

There are a variety of ways that you can get your CPD questions answered, so don't worry if you are feeling daunted by the thought of getting answers to so many questions. Many departments or units within the healthcare sector employ staff who have specific responsibility for promoting professional development and are recognised as experts in their roles. They work very closely with CPD education providers so they are very knowledgeable about what is on offer and can advise you accordingly. Increasingly, most CPD education providers also have a dedicated team of academics who often have nursing backgrounds who provide excellent links with the healthcare sector and are able to answer most (if not all) questions about CPD, thus helping you make the right choice for you. The links between education providers and the healthcare sector, as purchasers of CPD, are therefore robust and often include the specific commissioning of modules or units of study which have been identified as clinically and educationally needed in order to maintain the quality of healthcare delivery which is current and based on best evidence.

Your choices might be based on achieving a degree to attain graduate status or combining this with a kitemark award in your speciality or just finding out what qualifications and credits from previous study you have as part of your overall educational portfolio.

Are the courses delivered in ways which suit you?

When considering a specific CPD course your priorities may well be linked to how you access individual modules or units of study. You may find distance learning to be your favoured approach to learning. Along with this you a have a busy role at work and a family and social life to consider – which will also influence your choice of CPD programmes. Flexibility is therefore likely to be a principal feature for you. (However, if you are like me then distance learning is quite possibly the worst approach, as I know that my learning style suits a more traditional, attendance, taught classroom method of delivery.)

One philosophy of learning is based on 'work-based learning' (Lemanski *et al.* 2011). An example of this would be how within your role at work you have been able to investigate issues concerning risk or governance of care. As part of this task you provide an assessed piece of work which 'counts for' credit – in effect credit for work-based activities.

How long do CPD courses take and what do they cost?

HEIs determine the maximum academic time in which you have to achieve a particular award. Each HEI may have a slightly different interpretation, and the length of time often differs between awards at undergraduate and postgraduate levels. The length of time will in most institutions provide you with the opportunity to undertake courses on a part-time basis, where you can accumulate modules/units of study and count them towards your ultimate award.

Students often want to know the following:

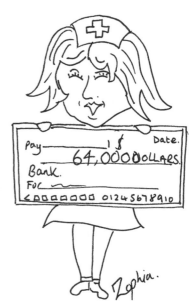

- How much does it cost?
- Who will pay?
- Can I pay bit by bit?

The 64,000 dollar question! The cost will vary, depending who the CPD courses are delivered by, how they are delivered and often whether they are credit-bearing or non-credit-bearing, for example.

Who will pay? This will vary. You may find that employers will pay for modules/units as they are integral to their strategic plan, or governance arrangements. You may also find that employers will pay and also provide study leave, which is the ideal. For some organisations there may be arrangements that fees will be paid but study leave will have to be negotiated (and may be within your own time).

Whatever the method of payment, it is essential that you know what it is, so that you do not get any unpleasant surprises.

In terms of credit-bearing degrees and postgraduate programmes, the educational providers will have varying arrangements on paying over the academic year. Some more enlightened employers will pay for you and arrange reimbursement from you via your monthly pay.

A major issue in payment is the changing nature of funding within HEIs for England (Department of Employment and Learning 2010). With the move towards a traditional three-year degree costing up to £9000 per year since 2013, some HEIs are considering whether CPD modules/units of study should reflect these changes and start changing their current costing models. In reality therefore it may cost as much as £1500 to gain the additional 120 credits to top-up a diploma qualification to a degree. This is calculated upon an assumption that each module to be studied would count as 20 credits and a total of six modules would need to be studied. If you divide £9000 (a full degree cost) by six this gives your 120-credit cost of £1500. However it must be remembered that this is just an example, and variations of module costs will be seen across the country and will be specific to individual HEIs.

The future remains uncertain as to the pricing point for CPD. What must be remembered is that CPD is not going to be immune from the wider HEI funding mechanism which sadly has the potential to negatively affect nurses' ability to fund CPD themselves, or indeed to gain funding from employers without some degree of contractual arrangement.

Summary

Nurses need to continuously update their knowledge and skills in order to maintain high quality evidence-based care and for them to demonstrate their ability to remain fit for practice and thus remain on the NMC register, as outlined in Chapter 10. Continuous professional development therefore remains and will continue to remain an integral and important part of healthcare. How CPD is delivered, what the subject matter is and the ultimate qualification for practitioners are only some of the facets to consider when considering a suitable path within CPD.

References

Betts, M. (2010) A Users Guide to Credit for Prior Learning through APCL and APEL. London: Linking London Lifelong Learning Network (accessed 17 March 2014).

Casey, D. and Egan, D. (2010) The use of professional portfolios and profiles for career enhancement. British Journal of Community Nursing, 15(11): 547–552.

Department for Employment and Learning (2010) Browne Report: Sustaining a Future of Higher Education: An Independent Review of Higher Education Funding and Student Finance, www.delni.gov.uk/browne-report-student-fees (accessed 17 March 2014).

Guy, E. (2006) The importance of Continuous Professional Development. Management in Practice, 2.

Lemanski, T., Mewis, R. and Overton, T. (2011) An Introduction to Work-Based Learning: A Physical Sciences Practice Guide. Hull: The Higher Education Academy.

Nursing and Midwifery Council (2011) The Prep Handbook. London: Nursing and Midwifery Council.

Royal College of Nursing (2010) Learning Zone. London: RCN Publishing, www.rcn.org.uk/_lz/index.php/cpdplan/index/prep/1 (accessed 28 February 2014).

Further reading

Cook, V., Daly, C. and Newman, M. (2012) *Work-Based Learning in Clinical Settings*. Oxford: Radcliffe Publishing.

Royal College of Nursing (2007) A *Joint Position Statement on Continuing Professional Development for Health and Social Care Practitioners*. London: Royal College of Nursing.

Useful web links

Chartered Institute of Personnel Development: www.cipd.co.uk/cpd/aboutcpd/

Royal College of Nursing: www.rcn.org.uk/development/practice/cpd_online_learning

Royal College of Nursing: www.rcn.org.uk/support/pay_and_conditions/agendaforchange/ksf.

Glossary

Academic Related to education and learning during programmes of study at educational institutions.

Accreditation of prior and experiential learning (APEL) A practice whereby credit is given to skills and experience obtained before starting a traditional training programme. It usually includes a collation of evidence in a portfolio which is often intended to permit an individual to gain access without the normal admission qualifications, or to permit exclusion from certain elements of a course.

Acute care The provision of emergency services which can be surgical or medical in nature, which often resolve following treatment and are usually of short duration.

Admissions tutor A person employed by the university (usually a member of the academic staff) who takes responsibility for overseeing the selection and recruitment of students on to university places.

Advanced practice registered nurse A registered nurse who is highly experienced and educated often to Master's degree level, able to diagnose and treat patients' health care needs or refer them on to a suitable specialist if required.

Attributes A selection of personal qualities, features and characteristics that people possess.

Autonomy The ability to work independently with an element of personal freedom in decision making.

Bursary A defined amount of money given to a student by an organisation (e.g. the NHS) to assist them in their pre-registration nurse studies. It does not have to be paid back.

Carer Somebody who takes care of a sick or aged person. This could be a relative, friend or neighbour.

Catheter A sterile plastic tube which can be passed into a person's body cavity to enable drainage of fluid – e.g. a urinary catheter passed into the bladder to drain urine.

Clinical Nursing or medical work or teaching that relates to the assessment, examination and treatment of people who are ill.

Clinical nurse specialist A nurse who has advanced clinical knowledge and skills in a defined area of nursing, e.g. renal, cardiac, orthopaedics, burns or accident and emergency.

Community care The delivery of care to people with a variety of health and social needs within a community setting instead of in hospitals.

Competence The ability to demonstrate a skill consistently and reliably to a defined standard.

Conduct The way in which people act or behave.

Continuous professional development (CPD) A range of learning events through which registered nurses are able to maintain, develop and demonstrate that they have the knowledge and skills to remain on the nursing register. Often referred to as continuous personal and professional development (CPPD).

Curriculum vitae A short description of a person's education, qualifications, and previous experience, most often supplied with job applications.

Defence The military forces (Army, Royal Navy, Royal Air Force) which protect a country.

Diplomats The term in nursing used to describe nurses who have obtained their registered nurse qualification following the completion of a diploma-level training programme.

Disability Physical or mental incapacity, which could be congenitally acquired or caused through injury or illness.

Disclosure and Barring Service (DBS) A government body which assists employers with making safe decisions linked to the recruitment of employees, in order to avoid inappropriate people working with vulnerable groups, including children.

Domains In the context of this book, domains are a defined range of knowledge and competence to be achieved during pre-registration nurse training.

Employability Having the right knowledge, skills, attributes and qualifications to be employed.

ePortfolio An electronic portfolio that consists of a collation of personal evidence of achievements.

Evidence-based Supported by applicable evidence from peer-reviewed research studies into clinical practice.

Family-centred care A model of care used by children's nurses which recognises the needs of the family rather than caring or treating the child in isolation.

Fees The payment required for students to access university courses, modules or programmes of study.

Graduates The term in nursing used to describe nurses who have obtained their registered nurse qualification following the completion of a degree-level training programme.

Health care assistant A member of the health care team who does not have a registered qualification and works under supervision of a registered nurse to perform delegated nursing tasks.

Health Care Professions Council A regulator which has been set up to protect the public. It maintains a register of health and care professionals (occupational therapists, physiotherapists and dieticians for example) who comply with their standards for their training, professional skills, behaviour and health.

Health Education England A special health authority of the National Health Service. It is responsible for the provision of national leadership and synchronisation for the education and training of the health and public health workforce within England.

Higher education Education delivered beyond high school at universities or similar educational institutions.

Higher education institution (HEI) An institution that provides courses that lead to higher education qualifications, including HNCs, HNDs, degrees, and postgraduate qualifications.

Holistic In nursing, relating to the care and treatment of the whole patient – taking account of mental, physical and social needs, as opposed to just treating an illness or disease.

Lay person A member of the public who has no relevant professional qualifications.

Learning difficulties Difficulties in the ability to attain and understand new knowledge and skills which can influence a person's ability to live an independent life.

Lifelong learning The process whereby knowledge and skills are obtained or enhanced throughout a person's life. In nursing this is linked to CPD.

Literacy The capacity to read and write.

Misconception A wrong or incorrect interpretation or view of something.

Misconduct Performance that falls short of what should professionally be shown by a registered nurse.

Module guide A document produced by an educational institution which provides all the information a student needs to study a given module of learning – e.g. the level of study, learning outcomes, dates of taught sessions, assessment strategy and reading lists.

Multidisciplinary team A group of professionals from different disciplines who work together to provide comprehensive assessment and care for patients.

Nasogastric Associated with the nasal passages and the stomach.

Numeracy The capacity to work with and understand numbers.

Nursing and Midwifery Council The statutory professional body that regulates nurses and midwives in the UK.

Objective structured clinical examinations (OSCE) A type of assessment of clinical competence in which students are introduced to scenarios under examination conditions and are required to demonstrate components of assessment and planning competence using an objective approach.

Person specification A collection of skills, qualities and qualifications that an employer determines are required for a particular job.

Plagiarism The taking of somebody else's work and passing it off as your own.

Post-registration education and practice (Prep) The professional requirement for nurses and midwives to demonstrate to the NMC in order for them to remain on the professional register.

Preceptorship The provision of support and guidance to newly qualified nurses and midwives in order to ease the transition from student to accountable practitioners.

Professional Someone who is a trained specialist in a particular area or occupation.

Reflection The art of looking back and learning from experiences.

Register An official list or record – for example, the register of nurses maintained and monitored by the NMC.

Royal College of Nursing A professional trade union for nurses.

Skill The practised ability to perform an action competently and reliably.

Tariff In education, the allocation of numerical points used for entry into higher education.

Transferability For knowledge and skills, the ability to be transferred from one area into another.

Universities & Colleges Admissions Service (UCAS) The UK organisation responsible for managing applications to higher education courses.

Visa An authorisation on a passport indicating that the owner is allowed to enter, leave, or stay for a specified period of time in a country.

Work-based learning Learning and training supplied by a university, college or other educational provider in the workplace.

Index